Body Dysmorphic Disorder

About the Authors

Sony Khemlani-Patel, PhD, is a licensed psychologist with over 20 years of experience in the treatment of obsessive-compulsive related disorders. She is clinical director of the Bio Behavioral Institute in Great Neck, NY, on the scientific and clinical advisory board of the International Obsessive Compulsive Disorder Foundation, and vice president of OCD New York. She has presented and published extensively in the areas of body dysmorphic and obsessive-compulsive related disorders and has co-authored two self-help books.

Fugen Neziroglu, PhD, ABPP, ABBP, is a board-certified behavior and cognitive psychologist and leading researcher in obsessive-compulsive related disorders. She is the co-founder and executive director of the Bio Behavioral Institute in Great Neck, NY, as well as clinical assistant professor at the Donald and Barbara Zucker School of Medicine at Hofstra/Northwell. She has published and presented over 175 papers in scientific journals and is the author and co-author of fifteen books which have been translated into many languages. She is on the scientific and clinical advisory board of the International Obsessive Compulsive Disorder Foundation, on the scientific council of the Anxiety and Depression Association of America, and president of OCD New York.

Advances in Psychotherapy – Evidence-Based Practice

Series Editor
Danny Wedding, PhD, MPH, Saybrook University, Oakland, CA

Associate Editors
Jonathan S. Comer, PhD, Professor of Psychology and Psychiatry, Director of Mental Health Interventions and Technology (MINT) Program, Center for Children and Families, Florida International University, Miami, FL
J. Kim Penberthy, PhD, ABPP, Professor of Psychiatry & Neurobehavioral Sciences, University of Virginia, Charlottesville, VA
Kenneth E. Freedland, PhD, Professor of Psychiatry and Psychology, Washington University School of Medicine, St. Louis, MO
Linda C. Sobell, PhD, ABPP, Professor, Center for Psychological Studies, Nova Southeastern University, Ft. Lauderdale, FL

The basic objective of this series is to provide therapists with practical, evidence-based treatment guidance for the most common disorders seen in clinical practice – and to do so in a reader-friendly manner. Each book in the series is both a compact "how-to" reference on a particular disorder for use by professional clinicians in their daily work and an ideal educational resource for students as well as for practice-oriented continuing education.

The most important feature of the books is that they are practical and easy to use: All are structured similarly and all provide a compact and easy-to-follow guide to all aspects that are relevant in real-life practice. Tables, boxed clinical "pearls," marginal notes, and summary boxes assist orientation, while checklists provide tools for use in daily practice.

Continuing Education Credits

Psychologists and other healthcare providers may earn five continuing education credits for reading the books in the *Advances in Psychotherapy* series and taking a multiple-choice exam. This continuing education program is a partnership of Hogrefe Publishing and the National Register of Health Service Psychologists. Details are available at https://www.hogrefe.com/us/cenatreg

The National Register of Health Service Psychologists is approved by the American Psychological Association to sponsor continuing education for psychologists. The National Register maintains responsibility for this program and its content.

Advances in Psychotherapy – Evidence-Based Practice, Volume 44

Body Dysmorphic Disorder

Sony Khemlani-Patel
Bio Behavioral Institute, Great Neck, NY

Fugen Neziroglu
Bio Behavioral Institute, Great Neck, NY, and
Zucker School of Medicine at Hofstra/Northwell, Hempstead, NY

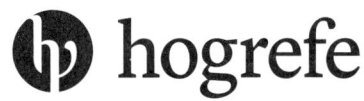

Library of Congress of Congress Cataloging in Publication information for the print version of this book is available via the Library of Congress Marc Database under the Library of Congress Control Number 2021948128

Library and Archives Canada Cataloguing in Publication
Title: Body dysmorphic disorder / Sony Khemlani-Patel (Bio Behavioral Institute, Great Neck, NY),
 Fugen Neziroglu (Bio Behavioral Institute, Great Neck, NY, and Zucker School of Medicine at
 Hofstra/Northwell, Hempstead, NY)
Names: Khemlani-Patel, Sony, author. | Neziroglu, Fugen A., 1951- author.
Series: Advances in psychotherapy--evidence-based practice ; v. 4.
Description: Series statement: Advances in Psychotherapy--Evidence-Based Practice ; volume 44 |
 Includes bibliographical references.
Identifiers: Canadiana (print) 20210339470 | Canadiana (ebook) 20210339519 | ISBN 9780889375000
 (softcover) | ISBN 9781616765002 (PDF) | ISBN 9781613345009 (EPUB)
Subjects: LCSH: Body dysmorphic disorder. | LCSH: Body dysmorphic disorder—Treatment.
Classification: LCC RC569.5.B64 K54 2021 | DDC 616.85/2—dc23

© 2022 by Hogrefe Publishing

www.hogrefe.com

The authors and publisher have made every effort to ensure that the information contained in this text is in accord with the current state of scientific knowledge, recommendations, and practice at the time of publication. In spite of this diligence, errors cannot be completely excluded. Also, due to changing regulations and continuing research, information may become outdated at any point. The authors and publisher disclaim any responsibility for any consequences which may follow from the use of information presented in this book.

Registered trademarks are not noted specifically as such in this publication. The use of descriptive names, registered names, and trademarks does not imply, even in the absence of a specific statement, that such names are exempt from the relevant protective laws and regulations and therefore free for general use.

Cover image: © stock_colors – iStock.com

PUBLISHING OFFICES

USA:	Hogrefe Publishing Corporation, 361 Newbury Street, 5th Floor, Boston, MA 02115
	Phone (857) 880-2002; E-mail customerservice@hogrefe.com
EUROPE:	Hogrefe Publishing GmbH, Merkelstr. 3, 37085 Göttingen, Germany
	Phone +49 551 99950-0, Fax +49 551 99950-111; E-mail publishing@hogrefe.com

SALES & DISTRIBUTION

USA:	Hogrefe Publishing, Customer Services Department,
	30 Amberwood Parkway, Ashland, OH 44805
	Phone (800) 228-3749, Fax (419) 281-6883; E-mail customerservice@hogrefe.com
UK:	Hogrefe Publishing, c/o Marston Book Services Ltd., 160 Eastern Ave.,
	Milton Park, Abingdon, OX14 4SB
	Phone +44 1235 465577, Fax +44 1235 465556; E-mail direct.orders@marston.co.uk
EUROPE:	Hogrefe Publishing, Merkelstr. 3, 37085 Göttingen, Germany
	Phone +49 551 99950-0, Fax +49 551 99950-111; E-mail publishing@hogrefe.com

OTHER OFFICES

CANADA:	Hogrefe Publishing Corporation, 82 Laird Drive, East York, Ontario M4G 3V1
SWITZERLAND:	Hogrefe Publishing, Länggass-Strasse 76, 3012 Bern

No part of this book may be reproduced, stored in a retrieval system or transmitted, in any form or by any means, electronic, mechanical, photocopying, microfilming, recording or otherwise, without written permission from the publisher.

Printed and bound in the USA

ISBN 978-0-88937-500-0 (print) • ISBN 978-1-61676-500-2 (PDF) • ISBN 978-1-61334-500-9 (EPUB)
https://doi.org/10.1027/00500-000

Contents

1	**Description**	1
1.1	Terminology	1
1.2	History	1
1.3	Obsessive-Compulsive and Related Disorders	2
1.4	Definition	2
1.4.1	Specifiers	2
1.4.2	Insight	2
1.5	Normal Concerns Versus BDD	3
1.6	Symptomatology	3
1.7	Epidemiology	5
1.8	Gender Differences	5
1.9	Onset, Course, and Prognosis	6
1.10	Functional Impairment	6
1.11	Suicidality	6
1.12	Quality of Life	7
1.13	Comorbidity and Differential Diagnosis	7
1.13.1	Depression	7
1.13.2	Social Anxiety	7
1.13.3	Obsessive-Compulsive Disorder	8
1.13.4	Personality Disorders	8
1.13.5	Anorexia Nervosa	9
1.13.6	Excoriation Disorder (Skin Picking)	9
1.13.7	Olfactory Reference Syndrome	10
1.14	Teasing and Bullying	10
1.15	History of Abuse	10
1.16	Diagnostic Procedures and Documentation	11
1.16.1	Diagnostic Interviews	11
1.16.2	Symptom Severity Measures	11
1.16.3	Insight Measures	12
1.17	Summary	12
2	**Theories and Models**	14
2.1	Biological Theories	14
2.1.1	Neurochemical Theories	14
2.1.2	Neuroanatomical Theories	15
2.1.3	Neuropsychological Models	16
2.2	Psychological Theories	16
2.2.1	Evolutionary Theory	16
2.2.2	Learning Theory	17
2.2.3	Cognitive Behavior Model Based on Social Learning	17
2.2.4	The Self as an Aesthetic Object	21
2.3	Summary	23

3	**Diagnosis and Treatment Indications**	24
3.1	Therapist Variables in Initial Sessions	24
3.2	Diagnostic Assessment	25
3.2.1	Connection Between Preoccupation and Compulsive and Avoidance Behaviors	26
3.2.2	Typical Day	26
3.3	Factors That Influence Treatment	27
3.3.1	Overvalued Ideation	27
3.3.2	Demographic Variables	27
3.3.3	Comorbidity	28
3.3.4	Previous Treatment Experience	28
3.4	Addressing Need for Cosmetic Surgery	28
3.5	Establishing Treatment Goals	29
3.6	Identifying the Appropriate Treatment	30
3.6.1	Medication for BDD	30
3.6.2	Cognitive Behavior Therapy for BDD	31
3.7	Summary	31
4	**Treatment**	**32**
4.1	Methods of Treatment	32
4.1.1	Assessment	32
4.1.2	Psychoeducation	35
4.1.3	Treatment Orientation and Engagement	36
4.1.4	Cognitive Therapy	38
4.1.5	Exposure and Response Prevention	40
4.1.6	Perceptual Retraining	45
4.2	Mechanisms of Action	47
4.3	Efficacy and Prognosis	48
4.4	Variations and Combinations of Methods	48
4.4.1	Attentional Training Technique and Task Concentration	49
4.4.2	Cognitive Remediation	51
4.4.3	Third Wave Therapies	52
4.4.4	Addressing Trauma and Loss	53
4.4.5	Addressing Skin Picking and Hair Pulling	55
4.4.6	Self-Surgery	57
4.4.7	Addressing Poor Quality of Life	57
4.4.8	Maintenance and Relapse Prevention	57
4.5	Problems Carrying Out the Treatments	58
4.5.1	Addressing Desire for Cosmetic Surgery	58
4.5.2	Addressing Suicidality	60
4.5.3	Nonadherence to Treatment	60
4.5.4	Family Involvement and Accommodation	61
4.6	Multicultural Issues in Treatment	61
4.7	Summary	62

5	**Case Vignettes**	63
5.1	Case Vignette 1: Post Accident Preoccupation With Nose	63
5.2	Case Vignette 2: Preoccupation With Facial Shape and Muscle Dysmorphia	68
5.3	Case Vignette 3: Preoccupation With Skin Accompanied by Skin Picking	73
6	**Further Reading**	78
7	**References**	79
8	**Appendix: Tools and Resources**	90

1

Description

1.1 Terminology

Body dysmorphic disorder (BDD), previously considered a somatoform disorder, was incorporated into the newly established *obsessive-compulsive and related disorders* (OCRDs) in the 5th edition of the *Diagnostic and Statistical Manual of Mental Disorders* (DSM-5; American Psychiatric Association, 2013). This category consists of disorders characterized by intrusive thoughts (obsessions) or repetitive behaviors (compulsions) (see Section 1.3).

1.2 History

BDD (referred to then as "dysmorphophobia") first appeared in the DSM in the 3rd edition (DSM-III; American Psychiatric Association, 1980) as an "atypical somatoform disorder." Diagnostic criteria were not included, resulting in minimal attention in the psychiatric literature.

With the publication of the DSM-III-R (American Psychiatric Association, 1987), BDD was established with diagnostic criteria as a "somatoform disorder," and the term was changed to "body dysmorphic disorder." No changes occurred in the publication of DSM-IV and DSM-IV-TR. The current DSM-5 diagnostic criteria are more detailed, reflecting the increase in recognition and research. The criteria include specifiers including insight levels.

BDD first appeared in the psychiatric literature in 1891, with the publication of a paper by an Italian psychiatrist Enrico Morselli. He coined the term "dysmorphophobia," noting the desperation and intensity of the fear and thoughts (Morselli, 1891). Other European psychiatrists, including Pierre Janet, Emil Kraepelin, and most famously Sigmund Freud, have published case histories of BDD patients. Freud's Wolf Man was a Russian aristocrat who had a preoccupation with the shape of his nose, accompanied by frequent mirror checking. He carried a small mirror in his pocket, checked for pores, and powdered his nose multiple times a day. His nickname came from recurrent dreams of wolves staring at him. He was later treated by one of Freud's protégées, Ruth Brunswick, who published a paper in 1928 describing his symptoms in detail (Brunswick, 1928).

The disorder was largely unknown until the *OCD spectrum* of related disorders became a model for conceptualization and treatment, leading to the official classification of obsessive-compulsive and related disorders in 2013.

1.3 Obsessive-Compulsive and Related Disorders

The *obsessive-compulsive and related disorders* (OCRDs) category was established with the 2013 publication of the DSM-5. This category designates disorders characterized by obsessions and/or compulsions. Obsessions are defined as intrusive, repetitive, and persistent thoughts that cause distress. Compulsions are repetitive behaviors or mental acts that are excessive, ritualistic, and repetitive. In addition to *obsessive-compulsive disorder* (OCD), BDD, and *trichotillomania*, this category includes the newly established *hoarding disorder* and *excoriation disorder* (skin picking).

> BDD is an obsessive-compulsive and related disorder

The existing literature had established overlapping features, referring to this cluster as the "obsessive-compulsive spectrum disorders." Similarities in symptom profile, treatment response, and comorbidity supported the categorization (Hollander et al., 2007).

1.4 Definition

BDD is characterized by a preoccupation with one or more perceived defects or flaws in physical appearance that are not observable to others or may appear slight to others. At some point the individual with BDD has engaged in repetitive behaviors, such as mirror checking, excessive grooming, skin picking, or seeking reassurance from others, or mental acts such as comparing appearance to that of others.

1.4.1 Specifiers

DSM-5 describes *muscle dysmorphia* as a specifier for BDD. This form of BDD is a preoccupation with the idea that one's "body build is too small or insufficiently muscular" (American Psychiatric Association, 2013, p. 243). Higher percentages of men than women are found to suffer from muscle dysmorphia. Common compulsions include excessive use of natural supplements and protein shakes to enhance exercise for muscle building, excessive exercising, use of steroids, seeking medical procedures to enhance body build, and specialized diets or food regimes. Clothing to either hide or enhance muscles is commonly seen.

1.4.2 Insight

> BDD individuals typically demonstrate poor insight

Insight as a further BDD specifier includes three categories: good or fair, with poor insight, or absent insight/delusional beliefs. Much research supports the fact that individuals with BDD demonstrate poorer insight than those with OCD (de Leon et al., 1989; Eisen et al., 2004; McKenna, 1984; Phillips et al., 2012; Vitiello & de Leon, 1990). In fact, appearance-related beliefs appear delusional at times, with up to 75% of patients showing lifetime prevalence of delusions. Referential thinking is frequently observed – believing that others are taking special notice of one's appearance or, specifically, one's "flaws" (Phillips, 2004; Phillips et al., 1994). Studies have found that BDD individuals misperceive others facial expressions in self-referent scenarios (Buhlmann et al., 2006). Poor to absent insight interferes with treatment engagement, necessitating the addition of therapeutic intervention, including motivational interviewing, clarifying treatment goals, and values-based exercises which will be discussed in Chapter 3 and 4.

1.5 Normal Concerns Versus BDD

Body image focus and discontent is common both in nonclinical and clinical populations, including in patients with depression and eating disorders. Worry, dissatisfaction, poor self-esteem, and depression are also evident in dermatological or medical populations, in which physical appearance is altered, such as in those with vitiligo, psoriasis, or scars.

Percentages of body image dissatisfaction in nonclinical samples are high, with more than half of the general population endorsing discontent with aspects of their appearance, and rates are continually on the rise (Garner, 1997). Body image is an issue that is by no means limited to women, with men experiencing poor body image at high rates as well (Adams et al., 2005; McCabe & Ricciardelli, 2004). Women tend to be slightly less anxious about appearance as they age, although body dissatisfaction stays surprisingly stable across the lifespan in adulthood until they are quite elderly (Tiggemann, 2004). Research across cultures suggests that while the definition of attractiveness may vary across countries, body image dissatisfaction and the desire for cosmetic surgery is found around the world, including China, India, Brazil, Italy, Greece, and South Korea.

Distinguishing BDD from normal concerns may at first seem daunting, but careful assessment of current functioning, daily behavioral patterns, psychosocial history, thought processes, and clinical history will ensure a proper diagnosis.

1.6 Symptomatology

Individuals with BDD can become preoccupied with any aspect of their physical appearance. Typically, one or two main body areas are the primary source of distress, but dissatisfaction with multiple areas is common (Neziroglu & Yaryura-Tobias, 1993; Phillips, 2005). Facial features are the most frequently cited area of concern, including skin, nose size, and hair (Phillips, 2005; Veale, Boocock et al., 1996). Often patients describe the flaw in great detail, such as size, texture, color, proportion to other body parts, and structural symmetry. At times, individuals describe dissatisfaction with their overall appearance, expressing a general disgust or feeling ugly and unattractive. This would still be considered BDD.

The hallmark of BDD is the level of distressing appearance-related obsessions, typically consuming many hours in a day. Thought content may consist of a focus on finding ways to improve or camouflage appearance, concern with others' perceptions, or hopelessness about their future if their appearance does not improve.

Repetitive and excessive behaviors aimed at scrutinizing, improving, or hiding the body part of concern are found in almost all individuals with BDD. One of the most common behaviors is mirror checking, consisting of either frequent brief checks or lengthy episodes of standing in front of a mirror. Any shiny or reflective surface is used to check their appearance; with individuals experiencing distress in brightly lit and mirrored public spaces. In some cases, avoidance of mirrors is common, and so is a vacillation between mirror checking and mirror avoidance.

> **Distress with specific body parts or general appearance can both occur in BDD**

Other behaviors very common to BDD include camouflaging and hiding the perceived defect, such as wearing hats to hide hair loss or excessive make-up application to cover acne. Comparing oneself with others has been found in up to 94% of individuals with BDD (Phillips, Menard et al., 2005). Social media images or magazine photos may be collected as sources of comparison. Some individuals will look at photographs of themselves at different time periods in their lives or use cellular phone cameras to evaluate appearance in different poses or lighting. Comparison with family members to assess similarities and differences can be driven by the desire to look alike or different from loved ones. Measuring one's body parts to compare them with a self-imposed standard or as a comparison with others is common as well.

Attempts to improve the body part may include extreme measures such as cosmetic or dermatological procedures or more self-initiated procedures, such as skin peels, frequent haircuts, teeth whitening, and other beauty-enhancing products related to the body part of concern.

Seeking reassurance can become a source of conflict with family members as loved ones can alternate between providing reassurance and becoming frustrated and antagonistic. Family members can misattribute BDD behaviors to vainness or self-absorption. Seeking compliments via indirect methods is also common, such as discussing topics related to beauty or appearance.

Avoidance of social and public situations occurs in varying degrees in almost all individuals with BDD. Avoidance of crowded or brightly lit places is quite common, as are situations involving a focus on appearance, such as bars and formal social events. Many BDD individuals vacillate between the desire to be noticed and the desire to hide. Many may avoid medical appointments, exercising, and activities involving outdoor activities.

Skin picking prevalence rates are alarmingly high in BDD; lifetime rates are approximately 45% (Grant et al., 2006). The skin picking creates further distress due to the resulting scars and a spiral of attempts to fix the damage due to the picking. The desire to achieve perfectly smooth skin leads to visual inspection as well as repeatedly feeling for bumps on body parts. The tactile experience can increase mirror checking and vice versa. In our clinical experience, the function of picking behavior evolves from appearance-based, to serving multiple other purposes, such as emotion regulation, further strengthening the behavior.

1.7 Epidemiology

To date, three large prevalence studies for BDD within the general population have been conducted – two in Germany and one in the US. Results were quite similar in all three, with reported prevalence rates of 1.7%, 1.8%, and 2.4% (Buhlmann et al., 2010; Koran et al., 2008; Rief et al, 2006). Gender distribution in these studies suggested a slightly higher prevalence for women than men. A general consensus in the field suggests a relatively equal gender distribution for BDD.

Rates vary, however, depending on the population studied. Within international and US college populations, rates appear to be higher, with a prevalence of 4.8% found in a Turkish college population (Cansever et al., 2003) and of 5.8% in Pakistani medical students (Taqui et al., 2008).

Within clinical populations, prevalence rates are higher than in the general population. In adult inpatient psychiatric settings, rates range from 13.1% to 16% (Conroy et al., 2008; Grant et al., 2001). BDD patients are unlikely to report their symptoms unless specifically asked to do so by mental health providers (Phillips, 2005). Rates in adolescent inpatient hospitals have been documented at 4.5% (Dyl et al., 2006).

Prevalence rates in dermatology and cosmetic surgery patients are high, as would be expected, with rates ranging from 7% to 15% (Castle et al., 2004; Conrado, 2009; Crerand et al., 2004; Kacar et al., 2014; Phillips et al., 2000).

Interestingly, one recent study found that prevalence rates of BDD in military personnel were significantly higher than in the general population, with rates of 13% in men and 21.7% in women (Campagna & Bowsher, 2016). The authors postulate that those with a preexisting emphasis on achieving an ideal body type may be influenced by that as a driving factor in enlisting. In addition, the significant attention toward physical fitness in the military may reinforce dysfunctional beliefs in those who are already predisposed.

> **BDD prevalence is approximately 2% in the general population**

> **BDD is found globally and has roughly equal gender distribution**

1.8 Gender Differences

Research has shown that BDD is found relatively equally in both genders, with studies citing similar clinical characteristics, age of onset, clinical course, demographics, impairment, and symptom severity (Phillips & Diaz, 1997). Skin and facial concerns are similar in both genders (Perugi et al., 1997; Phillips & Diaz, 1997). There are minor expected differences. For example, although both genders display concerns with hair, men are more concerned with thinning or balding, while women become concerned with other features of hair (Phillips & Diaz, 1997). Women are likely to be more concerned with their hips and weight, while men are likely to be dissatisfied with body build and suffer from muscle dysmorphia at higher rates (Campagna & Bowsher, 2016). Genital concerns seem to be primarily associated with men (Perugi et al., 1997; Phillips & Diaz, 1997).

1.9 Onset, Course, and Prognosis

BDD has a chronic course and does not remit spontaneously

BDD typically has a chronic course. BDD onset is most frequently reported in adolescence, with a mean age of 16 (Phillips, 2005; Phillips, Menard et al., 2005). Appearance dislike occurs at earlier ages, but full diagnostic criteria are more likely to be met in mid to late adolescence. Longer duration of symptoms, being an adult, and severity level may impact remission rates (Phillips et al., 2006; Phillips et al., 2013; Phillips, Pagano, Menard, Fay, & Stout, 2005). Appropriate interventions can lead to promising outcomes. Left untreated, BDD does not typically improve spontaneously.

1.10 Functional Impairment

Individuals with BDD exhibit significant impairment across many domains of functioning. Work impairment is quite common with 39–53% of individuals being unemployed (Didie et al., 2008; Frare et al., 2004; Perugi et al., 1997; Veale et al., 1996). Many of those who do work struggle with regular attendance or are unable to maintain full-time employment. Attendance is often compromised due to the symptoms, such as mirror checking, morning grooming routines, as well as significant anxiety and distress about being seen by others. High depression rates can further impact functioning (Phillips et al., 2007).

Other domains of functioning are also affected. Up to 30% of individuals with BDD report being housebound due to the disorder (Phillips, 2005; Phillips, Didie et al., 2006; Rief et al., 2006). Psychiatric hospitalization rates are also high, with BDD being a significant reason for admission (Conroy et al., 2008). Social impairment is found to varying degrees in almost all sufferers. Between 50% and 90% of BDD individuals are not married (Frontenelle et al., 2006; Phillips, Menard et al., 2005; Veale et al., 1996), further supporting the evidence for avoidance of social and dating functioning. The level of functional impairment likely negatively impacts social support, financial status, occupational success, and subsequently overall quality of life.

1.11 Suicidality

Suicidality is a serious and concerning symptom in BDD and requires monitoring

Lifetime suicidal ideation is found in almost all individuals with BDD (approximately 80%), and attempts are alarmingly high at 24–28% (Phillips & Menard, 2006; Phillips, Coles et al., 2005; Veale et al., 1996). Completed suicide rates in BDD are 45 times higher than in the general population (Phillips & Menard, 2006). Comorbid depression predicts suicidal ideation, while posttraumatic stress, substance use, and disordered eating may increase suicide attempts. Level of functional impairment also predicts ideation and attempts. Shame may be a risk factor for suicide and depression (Weingarden, Renshaw, Wilhelm, et al., 2016). Suicide is a significant risk factor in this population and requires ongoing assessment and management. Suicide protocols may need to be incorporated into treatment delivery.

1.12 Quality of Life

Self-reported quality of life is lower for BDD than in many other clinical and medical populations, including those with depression, diabetes, and a history of myocardial infarction (Phillips, 2000). Given the high levels of functional impairment, overvalued ideation, and suicidality associated with BDD, it is understandable that quality of life is negatively impacted. Quality of life has been shown to improve with both cognitive behavior therapy (Khemlani-Patel et al., 2011) and medications (Phillips & Najjar, 2003; Phillips & Rasmussen, 2004). Treatment interventions for BDD may require a long-term plan beyond symptom reduction in order to develop life satisfaction. This may include career counseling, development of social and leisure activities, and strengthening of life skills.

1.13 Comorbidity and Differential Diagnosis

Comorbidities in BDD are the rule rather than the exception. The most commonly coexisting conditions are depression, social anxiety, and personality disorders.

Comorbidities are the rule, and depression is the most common coexisting disorder in BDD

1.13.1 Depression

Depression is the most commonly found coexisting disorder, with 53–81% of BDD patients presenting with comorbid major depressive disorder (Frare et al., 2004; Gunstad & Phillips, 2003; Phillips, Didie et al., 2006). Depression tends to develop after the emergence of BDD symptoms, underscoring the significant impact of the BDD diagnosis (Phillips, 2004). Clinicians often have to treat both conditions simultaneously, especially if the depressive symptoms interfere with ability to engage in treatment.

Many individuals with depression struggle with poor self-image, including low levels of appearance satisfaction. They may even endorse avoidance behaviors due to poor body image or engage in some mirror checking or avoidance. BDD should be considered as a separate diagnosis based on the level of primarily appearance-based thoughts and behaviors. In contrast, individuals with depression alone are likely to endorse dissatisfaction and general poor self-worth in multiple areas, with appearance being one area of discontent.

1.13.2 Social Anxiety

Approximately 30–40% of BDD individuals suffer from comorbid social anxiety disorder (Coles et al., 2006; Gunstad & Phillips, 2003), and 11% of social anxiety individuals suffer from BDD (Brawman-Mintzer et al., 1995). A dual diagnosis likely leads to more significant social avoidance than BDD alone.

Individuals with social anxiety overlap in their distress and fear of negative evaluation, and avoidance of public places and social interactions. The differentiating factor is the rationale for the distress and avoidance. Individuals with social anxiety are primarily concerned with being judged for their behavior, such as appearing anxious or boring. BDD individuals, on the other hand, are primarily preoccupied with how others will judge or notice their physical appearance.

1.13.3 Obsessive-Compulsive Disorder

Based on the closely similar categorization of BDD and OCD, comorbidity is to be expected. Due to the similarities, many studies rely on the comparison of the two disorders across a variety of dimensions. Comorbidity rates suggest that approximately 27–30% of those with BDD have a comorbid OCD (Frias et al., 2015; Gunstad & Phillips, 2003). The reverse rates are lower, with only 10% of OCD patients meeting criteria for BDD (Frias et al., 2015). When BDD is present in OCD, it tends to have a more negative clinical impact than the existence of OCD in BDD (Frias et al., 2015).

Differentiating the two conditions is based on the content of the obsessive worries, with OCD individuals worrying about harm to self, or exhibiting behaviors associated with distress, such as symmetry, just right feeling, or repetitive actions. Occasionally an individual with OCD may present with perfectionism related to appearance that on the surface may sound like BDD. For example, exhibiting significant distress with unnoticeable flaws in clothing, such as stains or dirt spots. This may be due to a desire to appear perfect or present oneself in a particular way. Typically, these appearance-based obsessions in OCD result from perfectionism or as a symptom of *obsessive-compulsive personality disorder* (OCPD). The differentiating factor is the lack of persistent beliefs about appearance flaws in the person with obsessive-compulsive symptoms.

1.13.4 Personality Disorders

The research investigating comorbidity of personality dimensions and BDD is scarce, although data suggest it is a common and crucial clinical variable. Studies based on previous versions of the DSM have found high percentages of comorbid personality disorders, ranging from 50 to over 70% of individuals. Cluster C personality disorders are most common, which include avoidant, dependent, and obsessive compulsive (Neziroglu et al., 1996; Phillips & McElroy, 2000). Personality traits include neuroticism, low self-esteem, introversion, unassertiveness, social anxiety, and inhibition, rejection sensitivity, and perfectionism (Hart & Niemiec, 2017; Phillips & McElroy, 2000). Despite the lack of data, clinicians frequently report that personality disorders reduce treatment adherence and possibly response.

1.13.5 Anorexia Nervosa

The presence of eating disorders in a BDD population is 32.5%, and the prevalence of comorbidity of BDD in *anorexia nervosa* (AN) has been found to be approximately 39% (Grant et al., 2001). Comorbidity requires addressing the disordered eating patterns as well as the core body image beliefs, and these patients may present as more severe and impaired, with higher risk for hospitalizations and for other comorbidities (Ruffolo et al., 2006).

Individuals with AN and BDD can be difficult to differentiate due to symptom similarities. Both experience body image distortion, obsessional thinking about appearance, and common rituals such as mirror checking, exercising, comparing self to others, and excessive dieting. Both may also become focused on similar aspects of appearance, such as overall body shape, stomach, and thighs. Preliminary neurological studies suggest that AN and BDD may also share similar abnormalities in visual processing including attention to detail, reduced processing of global features, and a focus on body parts of concern (Madsen et al., 2013).

The main difference between AN and BDD is the disordered eating patterns leading to clinically significant weight loss in AN. Although individuals with BDD may alter their diet and exercise excessively, they rarely restrict food intake to the degree seen in AN. In BDD, the focus is typically on facial features more than body weight and shape. If patients meet the criteria for disordered eating and weight loss as well as a primary focus on body weight, then a eating disorder is a more appropriate diagnosis.

BDD and eating disorders share many common features

1.13.6 Excoriation Disorder (Skin Picking)

Excoriation disorder is included as one of the OCD and related disorders. It is characterized by recurrent skin picking resulting in mild to severe damage to the skin. Comorbid rates are approximately 45% for lifetime skin picking and BDD (Grant et al., 2006). Comorbid skin picking occurs primarily in BDD individuals who are dissatisfied with facial blemishes, acne, or scars. The picking is engaged in to "improve" or remove the skin imperfections.

Individuals whose primary focus for skin picking is to remove or improve perceived or minor imperfections are likely suffering from BDD. Those with pure excoriation disorder will describe the behavior as a repetitive habit, triggered by feelings of anxiety, boredom, or an increased sense of tension followed by gratification, pleasure, or a sense of relief after the picking. Those with excoriation disorder may also suffer from other body-focused repetitive behaviors, such as hair pulling (trichotillomania) and cuticle biting.

It is important to note that in some cases of BDD skin picking, the behavior may eventually become habitual and serve secondary functions of self-soothing or anxiety relief from general daily stress. In these cases, treatment should focus on appropriate interventions for both BDD and skin picking.

1.13.7 Olfactory Reference Syndrome

Olfactory reference syndrome (ORS) is a lesser known psychiatric condition involving a preoccupation that one emits a foul or offensive body odor that is not perceived by others (DSM-5; American Psychiatric Association, 2013). Examples of concerns can include sweat, bad breath, foot odor, flatulence, or genital odor. Due to the lack of sufficient research, the disorder is listed in the DSM-5 as an example of an "other specified obsessive-compulsive and related disorder," rather than as a separate condition with full criteria. Individuals with ORS struggle with impaired functioning and engage in repetitive behaviors including excessive showering, use of cosmetic products to decrease the odor, smelling oneself, changing clothes frequently, and chewing gum (Pryse-Phillips, 1971). Avoidance of social, academic, or work environments is common. Suicidal ideation has been noted as well. ORS shares commonalities with social anxiety, OCD, BDD, and health anxiety (Feusner, Phillips, et al., 2010), but requires more research in order to be recognized as a distinct disorder in the DSM system.

1.14 Teasing and Bullying

A childhood history of teasing, bullying, and abuse may play a role in BDD

The research in childhood teasing and bullying suggests that the negative impact of these behaviors carries into adulthood and may influence the development of BDD psychopathology (Boyda & Shevlin, 2011; Buhlmann et al., 2007, 2011). Those with BDD report being teased about appearance and competency more often compared with same-age peers without BDD (Buhlmann et al., 2011). For those who attribute their BDD to a specific triggering event, teasing and bullying appear to be the most common triggers (Weingarden et al., 2017). In this study, those with bullying histories have been shown to have poorer psychosocial outcomes than BDD individuals with other triggering events. Elementary school children with emerging BDD are more likely to be both victims and perpetrators of bullying compared with same-age peers (Neziroglu et al., 2018). The preliminary research suggests that appearance-based teasing during childhood may be an important risk factor in the etiology and severity of BDD, influencing functional impairment and depression. Further research would clarify the impact, including longitudinal studies versus the existing self-report data, as well as to distinguish if those with BDD may have a social sensitivity to the perception of teasing or a possible bias in recall of childhood memories.

1.15 History of Abuse

Similar to teasing, abuse history is associated with functional impairment and adulthood psychological distress. Higher rates of sexual and emotional abuse histories have been found in BDD compared with OCD (Didie et al., 2006; Neziroglu, Khemlani-Patel, & Yaryura-Tobias, 2006). Disorder severity also may be associated with reported sexual history. A history of attempted suicide has been related to emotional, physical, and sexual abuse, suggesting that abuse history impacts BDD symptomatology (Didie et al., 2006).

1.16 Diagnostic Procedures and Documentation

This section reviews the empirically based self-report questionnaires and semistructured interviews to establish a BDD diagnosis and assess symptom severity. In addition to these BDD assessments, it is recommended that clinicians incorporate measures to evaluate depression, hopelessness, and suicidality.

Identifying BDD can be a straightforward process by asking about dissatisfaction, distress regarding the dissatisfaction, time spent on the preoccupation, including thoughts as well as related behaviors, and level of avoidance and functional impairment.

1.16.1 Diagnostic Interviews

The *Structured Clinical Interview for DSM-5* (SCID-5; First et al., 2015) is a semistructured diagnostic interview system with different versions that can be used in clinical practice, research, and clinical trials. With the publication of DSM-5, the SCID was updated to meet the new criteria. The Structured Clinical Interview for DSM-5 Research Version has an optional module for the obsessive-compulsive and related disorders that includes BDD.

The *Body Dysmorphic Disorder Questionnaire* (BDDQ; Phillips et al., 1995) is a brief self-report five-item screening measure that is easily administered and has high sensitivity and specificity. It is brief enough to be implemented in a variety of settings, such as inpatient psychiatric hospitals as well as cosmetic and dermatological practices. A follow-up diagnostic interview is recommended.

The *Body Dysmorphic Disorder Examination* (BDDE; Rosen & Reiter 1996; Rosen & Ramirez, 1998) has two versions; the original semistructured interview and a self-report version. The scale is designed for both diagnostic and severity measurement. It measures preoccupation, negative evaluations of appearance, self-consciousness, importance given to appearance in self-evaluation, avoidance, camouflaging, and checking behaviors. The scale is thorough, but takes considerable time to administer.

1.16.2 Symptom Severity Measures

The *Yale-Brown Obsessive Compulsive Scale Modified for Body Dsymorphic Disorder* (BDD-YBOCS; Phillips et al., 1997) is a well-established 12-item clinician-administered measure designed to assess BDD symptom severity over the course of the past week. The scale is based on the Yale-Brown Obsessive Compulsive Scale for OCD. The first five questions assess obsessional preoccupations about appearance, the next five measure repetitive appearance related behaviors. Item 11 assesses insight, and 12 assesses avoidance. Scores range from 0 to 48, with higher scores indicating more severe symptoms. In research, a cutoff score equal to or greater than 20 suggests the presence of a BDD diagnosis. A 30% decrease in BDD-YBOCS score corresponds well to a "much improved" categorization on the Clinical Global Impressions-Improvement Scale (CGI-I), while a 50% reduction corresponds to "very much improved."

The *Body Dysmorphic Disorder Symptom Scale* (BDD-SS; Wilhelm et al., 2016) is a self-report measure consisting of 54 symptoms divided into seven groups designed to assess the presence and severity of symptoms. The symptom groups are checking rituals, grooming rituals, shape or weight–related rituals, hair pulling or skin picking rituals, surgery or dermatology–seeking rituals, avoidance, and BDD-related cognitions. Patients endorse symptoms in the past week and rate the severity of those symptoms within the group. Two overall scores are generated by the measure: a severity score and a total number of symptoms score.

1.16.3 Insight Measures

The *Overvalued Ideas Scale* (OVIS; Neziroglu et al., 1999) is a 10-item clinician-administered scale that measures the level of overvalued beliefs in the past week. The patient, with the help of the clinician, identifies the belief to be rated. The scale can be used to measure multiple beliefs, with a score for each belief, and is applicable to other disorders such as OCD, hoarding disorders, and eating disorders. Each belief is measured on different domains, including the strength, reasonableness, accuracy, extent to which others share the belief, fluctuation, attribution, insight, and degree of resistance. Each question is rated on a 10-point scale, and a total score is calculated by averaging the responses, leading to a total score ranging from 1 to 10, with higher scores suggesting higher overvalued ideation.

The *Brown Assessment of Beliefs Scale* (BABS; Eisen et al., 1998) is a seven-item semistructured interview that also assesses the level of conviction and insight in beliefs, on a continuum of insight. The scale assesses beliefs on seven different dimensions including conviction, perception of others' view of belief, explanation of differing views, fixity of ideas, attempt to disprove beliefs, insight, and ideas of reference. The first six items are added to obtain a total score. Total scores can range from 0 to 24, with higher scores suggesting poorer insight.

1.17 Summary

BDD is an obsessive-compulsive related disorder categorized by a preoccupation with appearance either slight or not observable to others. Behaviors aimed at camouflaging or improving the body part of concern are found in almost all individuals. The complexity of the disorder is due to its associated poor insight levels, high degree of functional impairment, low quality of life, and high suicidal ideation and attempts. Comorbid conditions include depression, social anxiety, and OCD. Empirically based self-report and semistructured interview measures should be added to a standard clinical interview as well as measures for depression, hopelessness, and suicidality.

2

Theories and Models

A few theories have been proposed to explain the development and maintenance of body dysmorphic disorder (BDD). Although the biological research is limited, there are some preliminary neurochemical and neuroanatomical theories. This chapter will review established psychological learning theories, with an emphasis on the cognitive behavior model.

2.1 Biological Theories

2.1.1 Neurochemical Theories

Serotonin is thought to play a role in BDD etiology

Many of the biological models of BDD are derived from treatment responses to the class of medications called *selective serotonin reuptake inhibitors* (SSRIs), neuroimaging studies, and neuropsychological test findings. Etiology should not be inferred from any of these studies, and functional differences do not necessarily implicate neurological dysfunction as a causal factor. Most of the neurochemical theories of BDD are based on OCD research, because of BDD's similarity to OCD. In addition, similar to OCD, SSRIs are used to treat BDD, and therefore it is assumed that serotonin is involved in its etiology. However, there are relatively few randomized controlled studies exploring the efficacy of SSRIs. In one study, a serotonin reuptake inhibitor (SRI; clomipramine) was compared with a norepinephrine reuptake inhibitor (NRI; desipramine) and was found to be superior (Hollander et al., 1999). Many anxiety disorders also respond to SRIs better than NRIs, and therefore this difference does not necessarily establish causation. However, there are case examples in the literature that implicate serotonin as a possible etiological factor. These cases suggest that a serotonin receptor agonist or serotonin receptor antagonist can reduce or increase symptoms of BDD. The former involved the use of psilocybin (Hanes, 1996), and the latter chlorophenylpiperazine (m-CPP; Hollander & Wong, 1995) and cyproheptadine (Craven & Rodin, 1987). In another study, 5-hydroxytryptophan, a precursor of serotonin, led to an exacerbation of symptoms (Barr et al., 1992). However, again neither depletion of tryptophan nor use of serotonergic receptor antagonists, both of which increase BDD symptoms, are sufficient to indicate that serotonin is implicated in the etiology of BDD. A wide variety of other psychiatric symptoms also show a response to alterations in serotonin.

2.1.2 Neuroanatomical Theories

The area of the brain known as the *extrastriate body area* (EBA) is involved in the perception of the body, body parts, and its actions. BDD, a disturbance in body image, thus involves the EBA, which is located at the posterior inferior temporal sulcus/middle temporal gyrus (Downing et al., 2001) and the fusiform body area (FBA) found ventrally in the fusiform gyrus (Peelen & Downing, 2005). Neuroimaging studies should also look into the inferior occipital gyrus, left fusiform gyrus, superior temporal sulcus, hippocampus, amygdala, right inferior frontal gyrus, and orbitofrontal cortex (especially in the right hemisphere), areas involved in emotional reaction to the face (McCurdy-McKinnon & Feusner, 2017; Veale & Neziroglu, 2010).

It has been suggested that the EBA and the FBA can be functionally dissociated, with a more selective activation for local body parts in the EBA relative to more holistic images of the human body in the FBA (Taylor et al., 2007). The EBA and FBA are two brain regions of the extrastriate visual cortex that are highly sensitive to the perception of human bodies and body parts. Functional magnetic resonance imaging (fMRI) demonstrates significant activation in both the EBA and FBA in response to body and body parts stimuli visually presented in different formats such as photos, line drawings, stick figures, and silhouettes, compared with control stimuli such as faces and face parts, tools and tool parts, and landscapes (Downing et al., 2001; Peelen & Downing, 2005; Schwarzlose et al., 2005; Spiridon et al., 2006; Weiner & Grill-Spector, 2010).

Neuroimaging studies have demonstrated that individuals with BDD, as compared with healthy controls, activate left hemisphere hyperactivity in response to normal and low spatial frequency images (Feusner, Townsend, Bystritsky, & Bookheimer, 2007). Controls activate the right hemisphere pattern in general and left hemisphere only when the faces contain high detail. In the studies, individuals with BDD activated left hemisphere hyperactivity regardless of whether the matching photographs of other people's faces contained high or low detail. In other words, it seems BDD patients were attempting to extract details even when there were none. Several fMRI studies (Feusner et al., 2009) have illustrated lower-than-average activity in the visual cortex regarding low spatial frequency images involving either their own face or the faces of others. Overall, BDD individuals demonstrated imbalances in global versus local or detail visual processing. This abnormality was not only evidenced in faces but also in non-face objects as well. In addition, the amygdala was highly activated for both the low and high spatial frequency images suggesting a heightened emotional response for faces. Activity in the amygdala may lead to emotional arousal (e.g., anxiety), which is positively associated with activity in the ventral visual stream, suggesting that the symptoms of anxiety in BDD might affect activity in ventral visual systems that are responsible for enhanced detailed visual processing. Anxiety might also heighten perceptual distortions in BDD. Alternatively, greater activity in the ventral visual stream might increase anxiety.

In summary, most neuroimaging studies of visual processing have suggested deficiencies in global and configural visual processing. These imbalances in

> BDD may involve deficits in global and configural visual processing

global versus local processing may explain why individuals with BDD detect "flaws." They are unable to see the flaw within the context of the whole.

2.1.3 Neuropsychological Models

The *Rey-Osterrieth Complex Figure* is a test of visuospatial construction and memory in which the individual is asked to look at and then draw a complex figure. Individuals with BDD recalled more details of the figure rather than the larger organizational features (Deckersbach et al., 2000; Sidali, 2018). The *Inverted Faces Task* also looks at holistic versus detailed visual processing (Feusner, Moller, et al., 2010). On this task, individuals are asked to pick the face that is the same as the one they previously saw in an upright or inverted orientation. The latter test is theorized to require detailed rather than holistic visual processing. Again, individuals with BDD exhibit problems with the inverted task when allowed to view it for a long time but not for a short duration (Feusner, Moller, et al., 2010). It may be that, similar to with mirror gazing, when they view something for a long time, they are encoding the details. The *Embedded Figures Task* also suggested more detailed versus global processing (Kerwin et al., 2014). A global processing defect was also studied looking at the ability to accurately identify emotional expressions in others. Individuals with BDD had significantly more errors in identifying emotional expressions, suggesting abnormalities in visual information processing.

2.2 Psychological Theories

The most prominent psychological theories are *evolutionary theory* and *learning theory*. The latter relies on a cognitive model, and some variations of that model have been provided by various researchers (Neziroglu, Roberts, & Yaryura-Tobias, 2004; Veale, 2010; Wilhelm, Phillips, & Steketee, 2013).

2.2.1 Evolutionary Theory

Evolutionary theory is based on the fact that evolution acts to promote reproductive success rather than to enhance the health of the species. Attractiveness may lead to more success in securing a mate, and there is significant literature on sexual attraction as it relates to body symmetry, which has been linked to reproductive health (Hart & Phillips, 2013). Almost 25% of BDD individuals report concerns with symmetry, such as a crooked nose, asymmetrical eyebrows, upper lip too thin in relation to lower lip, etc. Traits that are adaptive in some ways may be pathological when taken to an extreme. Grooming may be adaptive, but excess use of it, as in BDD, may be maladaptive. Body image concerns, rather than BDD per se, may explain the evolutionary theory of behaviors leading to attraction of a reproductively healthy mate.

2.2.2 Learning Theory

Learning theory is based on how individuals learn thoughts and behaviors and how they are maintained. Models have focused more on maintenance and triggers than on etiology. Veale (2004; Veale et al., 1996) and Neziroglu (2004) have proposed cognitive behavior models specific to BDD that incorporate several themes of Cash's cognitive learning social model of body image disturbance (Cash, 1997, 2002). The Cash model describes how societal, interpersonal, physical, and personality attributes all contribute to the development of body image perception. This perception, and the emotional consequences that come along with it, are strongly maintained through negative reinforcement. There are two different bases from which cognitive behavior theory can spring. Neziroglu and colleagues have emphasized a cognitive behavior model based on social learning and relational frame theory (Neziroglu, Roberts, & Yaryura-Tobias, 2004; Neziroglu, Khemlani-Patel, & Veale, 2008). Veale and colleagues, however, have proposed a model based on the self as an aesthetic object (Baldock & Veale, 2017; Veale, 2004).

2.2.3 Cognitive Behavior Model Based on Social Learning

Biological Predisposition
In Figure 1, "biological predisposition" refers to the diathesis-stress model in which an individual has to have a certain biological predisposition to developing a disorder. These factors can be neuroanatomical or neurochemical, or reflect genetic vulnerabilities.

Childhood Operant Conditioning
In Figure 1, "operant conditioning" refers to what a child experiences early on in life, which can play a crucial role in the development of BDD. When interviewing individuals with a BDD diagnosis, Neziroglu and colleagues found that appearance was highly reinforced during these early, salient periods (Neziroglu et al., 2009). If not reinforced during childhood, many of these individuals were reinforced at some point during their adolescence, for attention to their appearance, either to a particular body part or their general attractiveness. This reinforcement process solidifies the belief that appearance is the most important personal characteristic to the exclusion of behavior.

A CBT model explains the etiology and maintenance of BDD with neurobiological predisposition and environmental factors, including social learning and reinforcement.

The value system in which we examine physical attractiveness can stem from early, traumatic experiences, such as emotional and sexual abuse (Didie et al., 2006; Neziroglu et al., 2006) and bullying (Neziroglu et al., 2018). These traumatic events normalize the experience of negative affect. Later in life, this normalcy is replicated and reintroduced as the person observes their body (Cash et al., 1986; Osman et al., 2004; Rieves & Cash, 1996; Veale, 2004; Zimmerman & Mattia, 1999).

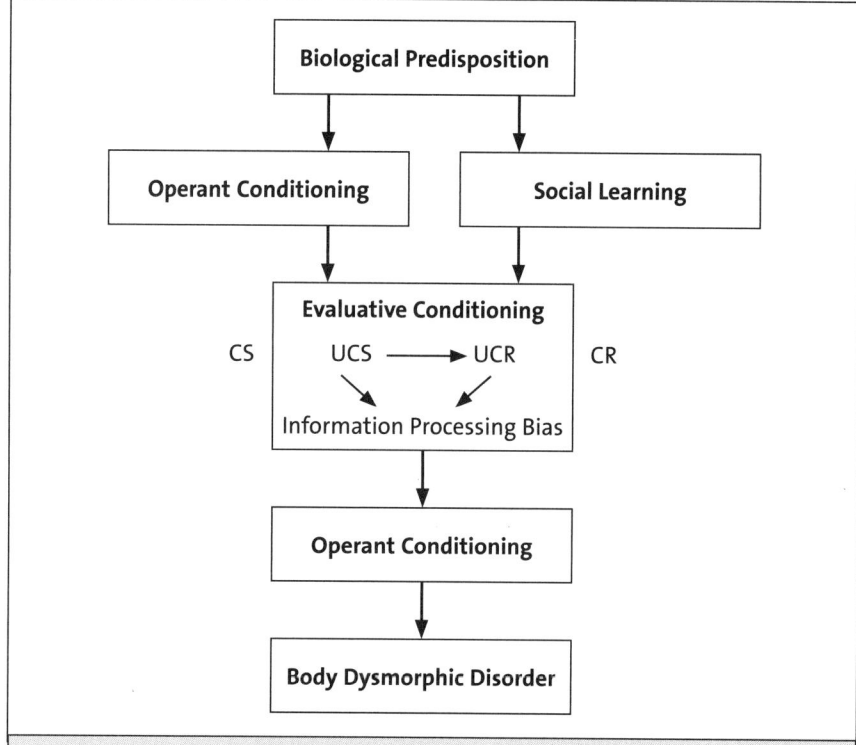

Figure 1
Cognitive therapy model based on evaluative and operant conditioning. Refer to the text for explanations of the different stages in the model. CR = conditioned response; CS = conditioned stimulus; UCR = unconditioned response; UCS = unconditioned stimulus.

Social Learning
In Figure 1, "social learning" refers to observing the reinforcement of beliefs and behaviors in other people, whether positive or negative, which can result in *vicarious learning* (Bandura, 1977). Vicarious learning of the importance of attractiveness can be affected by the sociocultural environment, with social media, social status, cultural body ideals, and the quest for physical perfection all playing a role. This vicarious learning can also be affected by one's closest social circles, such as immediate family and friends. In familial circles, the largest influential effect on learning is made through direct comments about eating, weight, and the body generally, rather than parental modeling of maladaptive behavior (Levine & Smolak, 2002).

Symptom Development Through Classical and Evaluative Conditioning
In Figure 1, just as classical conditioning utilizes physiological responses to reinforce or extinguish behavior, evaluative conditioning relies on the feelings toward a stimulus, such as liking or disliking, to fulfill the same function. Evaluative conditioning uses classical conditioning terminology to describe the pairing of two stimuli (unconditioned and conditioned) that results in a change of valence towards the stimuli (conditioned response).

The onset of BDD can be examined using evaluative conditioning terminology. The unconditioned stimulus (UCS) may be a negative or even traumatic incident(s) that surround one's physical appearance, for example, being bullied about one's appearance or actions. The unconditioned response (UCR), such as anxiety or shame, would then follow the UCS (traumatic incident). Eventually the UCS, the traumatic incident, becomes paired with a neutral stimulus (CS), one's physical appearance. Consequently, the UCR (anxiety or shame) becomes attached with the UCS (traumatic incident) and transfers to the CS (physical appearance).

Here is an example of evaluative conditioning for BDD onset. Your peers tease you about the size of your nose on multiple occasions (UCS), which makes you feel embarrassed (UCR). Following that consistently repeated event, you feel ashamed of anything associated with your nose, like a small bump that you previously haven't noticed or felt uncomfortable about (CS). Because the teasing is so unpleasant, anything associated with what you are being teased about also becomes unpleasant. Both the bump (CS) and someone's teasing you about your nose (UCS) become associated and take on the same negative connotation, and therefore elicit the same embarrassment response (i.e., a CR).

There are several factors that contribute to the onset and continuation of a disorder. First, biology plays a role, as some individuals are more susceptible to develop BDD than others. Second, experiences in early childhood, as illustrated and mapped out above, provide the learning history that connects one's physical appearance with negative affect. Finally, social learning is necessary, as the experiences of childhood need to be reinforced, either by external or internal factors, for BDD to continue. While these are common experiences of those who develop BDD, it will not be true for everyone. So, a diathesis–stress model would be important to explain any similarities between those who have and have not met these requirements but still meet the diagnostic criteria for BDD.

Information Processing and Development of Belief System Based on Relational Frame Theory

Because humans can think and rationalize thought, classical conditioning works differently for us than for animals. We also have a verbal language, and that likely contributes to the conditioning process. Humans can learn without direct experience; we can form bidirectional relations (i.e., we know what a barn is, without actually seeing a barn, and we can associate horses with barns). This ability to think in relations allows us to make predictions, but also gives rise to other relations. This is the basis of *relational frame theory*, which seeks to explain the associations we can draw through language and cognition, drawing upon both classical and operant conditioning to explain certain thoughts and emotions.

Language allows for the speaker to construct subjective connections between words. This is what allows a person with BDD to expand the disgust (UCR) that they felt when they noticed he had a pimple (UCS). The feeling of disgust (UCR) can be expanded to similar dermatological problems that everyone experiences. However, while acne and blemishes are not exactly the same thing, to someone with BDD, they evoke the same response. In fact, the same disgust response that this person has for their pimples can be felt when they interact with events or words that remind them of similar situations. The arbitrary nature of our language allows an individual to make these subjective connections, regardless of whether they are true or not. For example, someone in the situation described above may connect social success with blemish-free skin.

> **Relational frame theory describes how language contributes to evaluative conditioning**

Though children are not necessarily taught each relationship between events, as early as age 22–27 months they can understand these interrelations (Lipkens et al., 1993). Early in life, events that occur together or that are associated with past events can be arbitrarily related to each other through cognitive processes. This may occur through direct relation of the UCS and the CS, or through the interference of language. Beliefs introduced early in life are consistently reinforced as information is processed. During this time, attention is also refocused on the body part deemed defective; this process is enhanced through selective attention and therefore results in a stronger association with beliefs via the conditioning process.

Information Processing Research in BDD

The biased manner in which individuals perceive, interact with, and recall information in their immediate environment may contribute to the storage and recollection of adverse childhood experiences in adulthood. This misinterpretation can be seen in the results of several studies. BDD has been associated with hyperfocusing on details at the expense of the full image (Deckersbach et al., 2000) and selectively paying attention to stimuli, particularly BDD-related words, that evoke emotion (Buhlmann, McNally, et al., 2002). Finally, individuals with BDD are more likely then to misinterpret neutral social cues as threatening (Buhlmann et al., 2002). This inability to correctly assess social cues leads them to have more difficulty assessing the emotional facial expression of others and to believe that others are judging them disapprovingly (Buhlmann et al., 2004).

Higher Order Conditioning

Individuals with BDD are often more preoccupied with more than one body part. In fact, typically they are dissatisfied with up to three body parts, and one simply causes more distress than the others (Khemlani-Patel, 2001; Neziroglu et al., 2006; Phillips, 2005). This is best explained by higher order conditioning (the pairing of one CS with another CS so that they evoke the same response), which can occur directly or through relational framing. So, if someone is disgusted by their pimples, and generalizes a pimple to be any blemish, elevation on the skin, redness, etc., then any arbitrary facial abnormality can elicit the same disgust response.

Maintenance of Symptoms Through Operant Conditioning

Negative reinforcement, an operant conditioning principle, is known to maintain BDD symptomatology. Aversive emotions are reduced by avoiding them or seeking safety, which can manifest in behaviors like camouflaging, reassurance seeking, mirror checking or avoidance, excessive grooming, or avoiding social and public spaces. Engaging in these behaviors can reduce disgust, anxiety, and overall negative feelings.

Sometimes, an individual with BDD may like what they see in the mirror. This can be due to the random positive feedback they receive from looking in the mirror, which encourages them to keep checking the mirror. This kind of intermittent reinforcement is more resistant to extinction, which can prove trying during treatment.

The behavioral model of BDD discussed in Section 2.2.3, as developed by Neziroglu and colleagues, combines biological predisposition with early-life learning experiences (involving reinforcement of attractiveness and social learning). This pairing makes individuals more susceptible to classical and evaluative conditioning under these circumstances, eventually leading to BDD symptomatology. Relational frame theory may also help explain how certain thoughts and behaviors within BDD are elicited, as the associations between events depend on the learning experience of the person. All of these behaviors typical of a BDD diagnosis are maintained through negative reinforcement in order to reduce disgust, anxiety, and general negative emotive responses.

2.2.4 The Self as an Aesthetic Object

Individuals with BDD adopt the role of *self as an aesthetic object* as a result of self-focused attention. The acquisition of self-focused attention is a consequence of distorted mental images. It is hypothesized that this distortion of mental images is the result of intrusive thoughts and external events. There are four main components to this theory self as an aesthetic object: (a) mental imagery, (b) self-focused attention, (c) beliefs about the importance of self-focused attention, and (d) the lack of a self-serving bias.

> Mental imagery is central to the self as aesthetic object theory

(a) *Mental imagery.* Individuals with BDD often experience mental imagery or a "felt" impression of how they appear to others from an observer's perspective, making it central to the symptomatology (Osman et al., 2004). This drives future appraisals and responses, which is especially apparent in individuals with BDD and a comorbid social phobia. These individuals may use this "felt impression" of an observer to distance themselves from situations where their appearance may be potentially evaluated as negative, contributing to the maintenance of avoiding emotion.

(b) *Self-focused attention.* Two common responses to anxiety are orienting and defense, a sort of parallel to the fight-or-flight activation of the sympathetic nervous system. Orienting mode is characterized by scanning one's environment for possible threats in order to maximize potential responses to danger. This response can explain certain BDD behaviors, such as safety seeking or comparing, which are usually done to protect the individual from potential negative feelings (defense).

A hyperfocus on negative self-imagery and verbal association may prevent an individual with BDD from accurately appraising social situations, which could further confirm their fears of judgment. This may manifest as a lack of social skills, further isolating them and supporting those fears. Attentional resources may be so consumed with concern over these perceived negative evaluations that concentration may be negatively affected, and the individual may be unable to receive feedback about their appearance at all. Less severe cases may be more susceptible to feedback, which could facilitate more mirror-checking behaviors. This behavior, if performed for lengthy periods, can increase self-focus, and therefore feelings of "ugliness." If no mirror is available, this individual may use their self-image as an internal mirror to perform the checking behavior. In the presence of others or a mirror, an individual with BDD will begin appearance comparison processes by switching between their internal image and the appearance of someone else or their own self in the mirror, causing possible confusion about the way their appearance shifts.

(c) *Metacognitions about self-focused attention.* Little research currently exists examining the process by which beliefs surrounding self-focused attention form. From a clinical perspective, it is understood that a common motivation for individuals with BDD stems from examining their appearance and, more importantly, how others perceive their physical attractiveness. Often, their attention is focused on understanding the threat level of their current situation or, more specifically, if there is any possibility of humiliation or social rejection.

(d) *Self-serving bias.* When self-serving attention is directed by an individual with BDD at an external stimulus, either their physical body or an image, this is considered to be self-serving bias. Low levels of self-serving bias are associated with lower levels of perceived self-attractiveness. Research has identified that individuals with BDD are more sensitive to aesthetics when evaluating their own self-image (Lambrou et al., 2011). This pertinent sensitivity suggests that they may be accurate in body image perception, which runs concurrently with the self as an aesthetic object theory.

Negative Appraisal of Body Image

A distorted level of importance placed on body image leads to increased levels of negative body appraisal in those with BDD. In fact, appearance can become so strongly associated with the self, that it grows into the driving force behind a person's self-worth. A hyperfocus can be placed on social acceptance, symmetry, youth, or perfectionism. It is these values that reinforce the image of the self as an aesthetic or social object (Clark & Wells, 1995).

Rumination and Appearance Comparison

Evaluations and appraisals are manifestations of continued preoccupation and distress in those with BDD. They are commonly fueled by physical comparisons among others and rumination about one's distorted thoughts.

Appearance comparison. Individuals with BDD often compare their perceived defect to others, both those they know personally and celebrities. The development and maintenance of body image problems, not just BDD, is often perpetuated by appearance comparison (Heinberg et al., 1995; Stormer & Thompson, 1996). In BDD, the inability to construct an accurate view of how others view their appearance is caused by the prioritized attention given to specific features, instead of the body as a whole, as well as maladaptive mental images. These factors contribute to the overemphasized importance placed on physical appearance.

Rumination. Rumination, self-attacking, and worrying are common responses to intrusive thoughts, used by those with BDD. However, these responses do more harm than good. Rumination, in particular, becomes a feedback loop that perpetuates the preoccupation and distress through attempts to judge one's appearance while trying to solve incoming problems.

Emotions, Avoidance, and Safety Seeking

Avoidance safety-seeking behaviors often goes hand in hand with heightened negative emotions. Emotions in individuals with BDD are often specific to context and situation, but most commonly are ones of (1) internal shame in the face of physical comparison, (2) external shame and social anxiety, (3) depression, (4) anger and frustration, often directed at the self, and (5) guilt and shame. The most common functional purposes of avoidance or safety-seeking behaviors are (1) avoidance of thought and anxiety-provoking social situations, (2) altering appearance, (3) camouflaging, (4) distraction, and (5) reduction in negative emotions. Avoidance and safety seeking may give an individual a brief reprieve from the emotional aspects of body dysmorphia, but the reinforcement of these thoughts that these behaviors provide eventually increases them in the long run.

2.3 Summary

The cognitive behavior model of Neziroglu and Veale's self as aesthetic model both point to evidence that supports the development of body image beliefs and attitudes as influenced by experiences in childhood and social learning. Some of the overlapping examples of this include relationship with parents, friends, and family; teasing and/or bullying; and influences from the media. Another overlap between the models of Neziroglu and Veale are the attempted explanations of avoidance behaviors, negative emotions, and selective attentional biases. The only glaring difference between the two models is that Neziroglu and colleagues more strongly value the contributions that social conditioning and learning make to the development of BDD, while Veale and colleagues emphasize perceived observer's perspective, cognitive processes, and safety-seeking behaviors.

3

Diagnosis and Treatment Indications

This chapter will provide guidelines for assessment, treatment engagement, and treatment planning. Treatment of body dysmorphic disorder (BDD) requires a focused attention on developing and maintaining treatment engagement. Therapists need to establish a shared conceptualization of the target problem and treatment goals with their patient. Thorough assessment of suicidality and depression are also necessary in treatment planning.

3.1 Therapist Variables in Initial Sessions

Many BDD patients are reluctant to receive treatment and have poor insight regarding their perceived flaws. They may not have revealed the severity of their appearance preoccupation to professionals, resulting in improper treatment or insufficient progress due to a missed diagnosis. Patients may have instead received treatment for depression or social anxiety, but not BDD. Furthermore, patients' families are often the ones to enthusiastically seek treatment, while BDD patients are often reluctant or opposed to mental health services. Establishing a working relationship is critical to adherence, both in the beginning stages and as therapy progresses.

> **Credibility, flexibility, and BDD expertise help establish rapport and engagement.**

The therapist's approach from the first interaction is particularly important in treatment engagement, sometimes just to secure a second appointment. BDD expertise, credibility, and a flexible therapeutic style can aid in these early stages of therapy.

An initial evaluation should include a detailed gathering of day-to-day BDD symptoms. Asking thoughtful and specific questions about the level of preoccupation, the rituals, and level of avoidance communicates your expertise. If a patient has not been previously treated by a BDD expert, it is unlikely that another professional has conducted a similarly detailed assessment. Concentrating on the patient's area of concern is of utmost important to establish credibility. A willingness to understand their self-perception of their appearance in a genuine and interested way improves trust and engagement.

It is also important to allow the patient sufficient time to describe their appearance perceptions, and to respond in an interested and nonjudgmental manner. Demonstrating a true desire to understand the patient's appearance concerns also increases treatment commitment. It can be difficult to balance validation of the patient's experience while informing them of their BDD diagnosis, as they may see the diagnostic label as a dismissal of their concerns. While it is important not to engage in extensive debate about the diagnosis in early sessions, therapists can maintain their opinion on the reasons for their diagnosis. For example, the therapist could shift focus to the level of impairment and suffering about their appearance beliefs as a rationale for the diagnosis. Engagement usually occurs with a validation of the patient's suffering and need to restore functioning.

Even patients who are open to treatment may be extremely frightened to do so for many reasons. At times, they may be fearful to leave their homes for long periods of time or have difficulty in sustained interactions with others. Therapists can remedy these obstacles by being flexible in adjusting the office setting. Conducting a brief assessment of a patient's discomfort and making adjustments accordingly communicates your understanding of their daily struggles. This may include lowering the office lights, scheduling appointments when the waiting room is uncrowded, having them wait in the car or an empty room, or conducting some of your assessment via telephone, or a place where patients are most comfortable. Of course, this will be at the beginning of the engagement period and not a long-term therapeutic strategy. Most BDD patients may not have experienced that level of understanding or flexibility in other clinical settings or by family members.

Other suggestions for treatment engagement, establishing goals, and treatment planning will be provided later in this chapter.

3.2 Diagnostic Assessment

An initial *diagnostic assessment* will cover the patient's reason for seeking treatment, onset, history of symptoms, family response, cosmetic or dermatological interventions, psychosocial history, quality of life, medical history, family psychiatric history, and any substance use, as well as presence and history of trauma, abuse, and bullying. High-risk symptoms, strong conviction of beliefs, and patient's ambivalence often result in the necessity of using more than one session or longer appointments to complete a thorough evaluation.

Comorbidity is quite common (Gunstad & Phillips, 2003), so proper identification of all diagnoses is important. The order of treatment targets is guided by severity, high-risk symptoms, as well as symptoms interfering with treatment adherence and attendance. Reducing the interference of comorbidities can increase the effectiveness of the BDD treatment. For example, if a patient has past trauma and symptoms of posttraumatic stress disorder (PTSD), then those may require appropriate treatment before CBT for the BDD.

You can assess for primary versus secondary depression and social anxiety by gathering a history of the onset of symptoms. Patients may primarily avoid social situations for fear of appearance criticism. Their depression may be a result of appearance distress. Using the magic wand question is one clear way to communicate the difference to patients. Ask them, "If I had a magic wand and could take away your preoccupation and distress with your appearance, would you still be sufficiently depressed (or socially anxious) to seek treatment for it?" Patients are able to distinguish the difference with this line of reasoning.

Assessing overvalued ideation with the Overvalued Ideas Scale (Neziroglu et al., 1999) or the Brown Assessment of Beliefs Scale (Eisen et al., 1998) is a critical first step to determine the necessity of motivational interviewing and cognitive techniques in the treatment plan.

Using structured suicide measures such as the Beck Suicide Scale (Beck et al., 1979) will also guide treatment focus on reducing suicide risk via CBT suicide protocols. We believe that BDD exposure exercises are not recommended for patients with active suicide ideation.

The clinician can assess for readiness for change using the University of Rhode Island Change Assessment Scale (URICA) – Psychotherapy Version (McConnaughy et al., 1983) and determine if motivational interviewing techniques will be necessary to engage the patient in therapy.

Careful assessment is critical in treatment planning

Assessing for the patient's level of concern with the way they feel about their appearance versus their concern with others' view about their appearance is recommended. Most patients struggle with both, but may experience greater distress with one over the other. Distinguishing external versus internal shame can help the clinician to understand and develop a more thorough hierarchy. For example, patients who acknowledge that others do not take special notice of their appearance may not engage in the same type of avoidance as those who believe their perceived flaws are clearly observable to others.

3.2.1 Connection Between Preoccupation and Compulsive and Avoidance Behaviors

As in obsessive-compulsive disorder (OCD), establishing an understanding of the function of the avoidance and compulsive behaviors as they relate to appearance beliefs will help establish a thorough hierarchy. For example, is skin picking a function of dissatisfaction with blemishes on the skin? Is skin picking also a result of anxiety, boredom, or a need to self-soothe? Determining which behaviors are linked to which body part of concern aids in systematic behavior therapy exposure exercises.

Formal assessment measures given at the initial consultation can also be readministered to track treatment response and progress. Objective data to measure progress helps guide an evidenced-based treatment plan. In addition to the BDD-YBOCS and Beck Depression Inventory – Second Edition, it is helpful to screen for comorbid conditions and their severity, including hopelessness, suicidality, and perceived trauma.

3.2.2 Typical Day

Determining daily level of functioning, severity, and impairment can be conducted by asking a patient to describe a typical recent day, with details on how each activity is impacted by BDD thoughts, compulsive behaviors, and avoidance. For example, is their bathing and dressing routine impacted by their excessive use of the bathroom mirror or a grooming routine that often leads to tardiness and inconsistent work attendance? Is using public transportation a source of avoidance and distress? Gather details on a workday versus a weekend to help identify sources of distress and dysfunction. The typical day is used in two ways: as an initial diagnostic and severity measure and then later to gather specific behaviors and avoidance to help build a hierarchy. Hierarchy development will be discussed in Chapter 4 as a hierarchy method (see Developing a Hierarchy, in Section 4.1.4: Cognitive Behavior Therapy for BDD).

3.3 Factors That Influence Treatment

Treatment planning is most effective when consideration is given to the client's clinical presentation, cultural background, demographics, and previous treatment history.

3.3.1 Overvalued Ideation

Overvalued ideation (OVI) is likely the most challenging and interfering variable in treatment engagement and early assessment is highly recommended. Patients are unlikely to engage in treatment if they believe their suffering is a consequence of their physical flaws. Developing a shared conceptualization of the disorder as described below is necessary with high OVI. Treatment will progress at a slower pace allowing adequate time for rapport building, cognitive therapy, motivational interviewing, and psychiatric interventions. Exposure and response prevention exercises are less likely to result in the intended shift in learning. Patients with high OVI may not understand the purpose of the exposure exercise or come away from the experience with distorted conclusions. Previous beliefs may be solidified rather than challenged, so ERP should be delayed or adjusted to account for the degree of OVI. Chapter 4 provides specific suggestions on how to prepare the client for these exercises (see Section 4.1.4).

3.3.2 Demographic Variables

Age
BDD symptoms are similar across the life span and cognitive behavioral treatment is an effective strategy for all age groups. Clinicians may need to adjust the treatment to address stage of life stressors, such as declining physical health and loss in elderly patients. Body image focus may also be congruent with aging factors, such as hair loss and skin changes.

> Describe BDD as a preoccupation with appearance rather than as an imagined defect

Gender
BDD is found equally in both genders and treatment does not have to be adjusted based on gender alone. Body parts of concern may vary between genders, with men being more likely to be dissatisfied with body build. Symptoms overall are similar between the genders.

Ethnicity and Cultural Background

Clinicians will need to be sensitive and aware of how ethnic background impact's a person's beliefs and desire to seek mental health treatment. Family involvement also varies across ethnic groups. In BDD specifically, clinicians should pay adequate attention to cultural messages and standards of beauty.

3.3.3 Comorbidity

Comorbidity severity and interference determines if other conditions need to be treated concurrently or previous to the BDD. In most circumstances, depression is inherently connected to the BDD and can be simultaneously addressed. Clinicians should assess for depression related beliefs and address accordingly.

A personality disorder may need to be treated separately if clinically judged to be interfering with treatment engagement or adherence. Patients struggling with frequent interpersonal conflict or emotional dysregulation may need additional sessions to adequately address.

It may be prudent to separate out the treatment providers, with another clinician addressing the personality disorder especially if the patient could benefit from a Dialectical Behavior Therapy (DBT) protocol.

Suicidal ideation may also need to be addressed with evidence based protocols. See chapter 4 (see Section 4.5.2) for suggested suicidal treatment. Like depression, suicidality is often connected to the severity of BDD symptoms, thus the clinician may need to address both simultaneously.

3.3.4 Previous Treatment Experience

The secrecy and shame of BDD can lead to inadequate and incongruent treatment. At other times, patients have done a less formalized or partial trial of CBT. Gathering specific examples of past treatment experiences helps gear the most effective approach.

3.4 Addressing Need for Cosmetic Surgery

> The need for cosmetic surgery should be assessed early in therapy if your patient endorses intent

If the patient has been seeking cosmetic surgery interventions or plans to do so within a short period of time, this may become an early issue to address. Patients may enter treatment believing that if they engage in treatment and fail, then their families and treating professionals will support cosmetic surgery. Family members will go to great lengths to convince their loved one to engage in therapy, sometimes promising to pay for cosmetic procedures after therapy. If the patient's motivation for entering treatment is to prove its ineffectiveness, then the therapist has a very difficult road ahead. In this case, therapists will need to sensitively coach families to set limits on their role in supporting cosmetic surgery. We have encountered cases in which the patient frequently threatens suicide if cosmetic surgery is not possible, resulting in patients becoming oppositional and inconsistent in their appointments due to the family conflict, or canceling appointments at the last minute as a result of a dispute.

Here are some guidelines in addressing patient's desire for cosmetic surgery:

1. Incorporate family therapy to set limits and guidelines on cosmetic surgery conversations.
2. Therapists should share the research on the poor cosmetic surgery outcome in individuals excessively preoccupied with appearance. We acknowledge that some individuals are satisfied with surgery outcome, but this group has significant differences from those with BDD. They are not riddled with anxiety and depression and functional impairment. If a patient continues to be adamant about pursuing surgery, it is advisable to request waiting a few months to decrease anxiety, depression, and preoccupation. Therapists can also attempt to postpone the discussion of surgery for a later date.
3. Avoid initially suggesting that the goal of treatment is to change the patient's mind about cosmetic procedures. Keep an open mind and encourage the patient to tell you more about why they are seeking that particular cosmetic procedure.
4. Encourage the patient to improve their level of functioning in therapy regardless of their eventual decision to engage in surgery.
5. If possible, suggest a predetermined timeline to engage in therapy and delay the procedure.
6. If necessary, repeatedly remind patients about the negative outcome of surgery, especially if the patient suffers from an obsession with appearance.
7. Educate your patient that their presurgery expectation will influence their postsurgery satisfaction. Remind them of the risk of suicidality if they are not satisfied with the outcome. Discuss how perfectionistic expectations should be reduced before surgery.
8. Suggest and strongly encourage your patient to allow you to accompany them to any scheduled cosmetic surgery appointments to objectively hear the surgeon's opinion. Demonstrate that you do not have a prejudiced view of the necessity of the procedure, but would like to attend the appointment to hear the surgeon's unbiased opinion.

3.5 Establishing Treatment Goals

Therapists should directly discuss the patients' expectations and *goals for treatment*. BDD-based interventions should be delayed until clear goals can be established. Once you have established a mutually agreed upon definition of the disorder, goal setting is easier.

Initially, therapists can suggest that the distress, anxiety, depression, and daily suffering are important treatment targets. Therapists can also focus on the resulting impairment in daily life, such as social isolation, lack of dating or socializing, reduced work productivity, financial difficulties, decreased family engagement, and loss of leisure activities. Developing a plan to engage in these activities, despite the appearance concerns, can sometimes be an early engagement strategy. More than 80% of BDD patients struggle with depression, so this may also be an acceptable symptom to target if the patient is not ready to directly engage in BDD treatment. Behavioral activation actually leads to exposure and thus serves a double purpose.

Do not promise that treatment will help the patient see themselves as more attractive. This is not always achieved in treatment. Often, the patient learns to value appearance less and to accept that their view of themselves may not be accurate. There is usually a behavioral change in which functioning increases, suicidality and depression decrease, and perceptions are altered.

Exposure exercises for BDD are typically not incorporated in the beginning stages of treatment. Instead, therapists should focus on motivational interviewing for engagement, reducing some of the rituals gradually (including mirror checking), establishing a strong foundation in cognitive therapy, and attempting to improve daily functioning. Engagement often fluctuates, and therefore the therapist needs to be prepared to deal with reengaging with the patient at various stages of treatment.

3.6 Identifying the Appropriate Treatment

Empirically supported treatment for BDD is based on the long-established cognitive behavior therapy (CBT) and exposure and response prevention (ERP) model for OCD. BDD treatment outcome data support the efficacy of CBT as the foundation of interventions (Harrison et al., 2016). Pharmacological interventions consist of serotonin reuptake inhibitors (SRIs; Phillips, 2010).

3.6.1 Medication for BDD

SSRIs at higher doses are typically used in the treatment of BDD

SSRIs are broad-spectrum medications that have been shown to decrease BDD symptoms. To date, three double-blind placebo-controlled studies have supported the efficacy of escitalopram (Phillips et al., 2016) and fluoxetine (Phillips et al., 2002). A crossover trial demonstrated the efficacy of the tricyclic clomipramine (Hollander et al., 1999). Open-label trials of fluvoxamine (Phillips et al., 1998) and citalopram (Perugi et al., 1996; Phillips & Najjar, 2003) also showed improved BDD symptoms. Therapeutic doses for BDD are typically higher than necessary for depression, and at times exceed recommended dose guidelines. Augmentation with atypical neuroleptics is used in clinical practice, although research is scarce in this area. Due to the severity and chronic nature of BDD, it is recommended that patients maintain their medication regime for extended periods along with a maintenance course of therapy.

Medication noncompliance may be a problem in cases of delusional or highly overvalued BDD, because these patients do not believe a psychiatric intervention is appropriate for their physical problem. They may also be concerned that the medication will cause weight gain or acne, or otherwise negatively impact their appearance. Some patients have also expressed a reluctance to feel better with medications, as they feel this will dissuade them, or trick them into falsely accepting their appearance, and thus decrease their motivation for cosmetic interventions. Mental health providers must carefully assess for compliance and the reasons for noncompliance.

3.6.2 Cognitive Behavior Therapy for BDD

The treatment model for BDD is based on the similarities between OCD and BDD, as well as decades of rigorous OCD research demonstrating CBT and exposure and response prevention (ERP) as gold standards of intervention. Although more rigorous outcome studies are still needed, research to date has supported the effectiveness of CBT and ERP for BDD (Ipser et al., 2009; Prazeres et al., 2013; Williams et al., 2006). As phenomenological research data have emerged noting the distinct differences between the two disorders, existing interventions have appeared somewhat incomplete to address the severity and risk of patients who enter treatment. Clinicians, therefore, need to consider augmenting standard treatment with other empirically supported treatments to match complex symptom presentations, including suicide protocols, trauma interventions, family therapy, motivational techniques, and emotion dysregulation skills.

3.7 Summary

Early stages of treatment for BDD should consist of a systematic focus on engagement to ensure treatment adherence. Conducting an assessment of suicidality, comorbidities, overvalued ideation, and trauma are all important patient variables. Therapist style and expertise are critical in engagement. Therapists should demonstrate their expertise in BDD and be willing to be flexible in treatment delivery. Before directly targeting BDD symptoms, it is important to establish a shared definition of the problem in order to collaboratively develop treatment goals. If depression, trauma, and suicidality are impacting the treatment progress, then those symptoms may need to be addressed. The desire for cosmetic surgery can also impact on treatment engagement and may need to be addressed.

4

Treatment

BDD treatment typically involves multiple methods and approaches

The treatment for body dysmorphic disorder (BDD) has to encompass a comprehensive, multimodal, and flexible approach. This chapter will review guidelines and treatment interventions, which include standard cognitive behavior therapy (CBT), with additional techniques, including perceptual retraining, attentional training, acceptance and commitment therapy (ACT), and dialectical behavior therapy (DBT). This chapter also provides an introduction to modules as needed for motivation, suicidality, skin picking, and trauma. In many cases, BDD treatment length cannot be easily prescribed to a specific time frame or number of sessions. Typically, a more intensive approach with multiple sessions a week is recommended with a step down guided by the patient's treatment gains. Quality of life does not typically improve in the initial stages of change and requires ongoing sessions to build a meaningful life beyond symptom improvement.

4.1 Methods of Treatment

4.1.1 Assessment

Assessment should include the structured measures mentioned in Chapter 1 (Section 1.16) in addition to an evaluation of BDD symptoms. These should include the following:
1. Identify body parts of concern:
   a. Identify each body part of concern.
   b. Develop an understanding of what aspects of that body part are of concern, such as size, shape, texture, and so on. Ask what the patient actually sees in the mirror.
2. Identify obsessional thoughts and beliefs:
   a. Identify the content of the obsessional thinking. What does the patient think when they looks at themselves?
   b. Identify beliefs about the importance of appearance; how do they believe life would be made different by achieving their ideal looks.
   c. Identify the discrepancy between how others view them versus their own view of themselves.
   d. Determine the patient's worries about others' judgments versus their own judgment.
   e. Use a bell curve diagram to discuss the patient's rating of their current attractiveness versus their ideal goal (see Appendix 1). Patients

typically fall into two categories: those who believe they are very unattractive and desire to be in the average range and those who believe they are average or above average, but seek to be extremely attractive. It helps to differentiate the degree of importance they place on their body part of concern in judging their overall appearance. These factors can help in targeting core beliefs about perfectionism, inadequacy, over-importance of small details, and self-worth.
   f. On the bell curve, have patients indicate their rating of their overall attractiveness versus their body part of concern. Indicate to the patient that 68% of the population falls within the average range and that people get progressively more attractive or progressively less attractive. Refer to Appendix 1 for the bell curve exercise.
3. Identify avoidance and safety-seeking behaviors:
   a. For each body part, determine all of the ritualistic and avoidance behaviors that accompany it.
   b. What are the functions of each of the behaviors? Is it to improve, inspect, or camouflage appearance? Is the patient checking the mirror to magically wish that their appearance has improved since the last check, or do they seek reassurance that they are okay?

Typical Day Involving Assessment of Avoidance and Compulsive Behaviors

As mentioned in Chapter 3 (Section 3.2.2: Typical Day), asking a patient to envision a recent typical day helps confirm a diagnosis and assess disorder severity. The exercise can be revisited and expanded upon to gather more specific data on symptoms, triggers, cognitions, and level of interference. A typical day also helps gather a list of rituals and avoidances to build a hierarchy for exposure and response prevention (ERP).

The exercise is straightforward: Ask the patient to choose a day in the past week that represents their typical life and describe their activities from the moment they woke up and as they progressed throughout their day. Keep patients focused by asking, "What did you do after that…?" Pause the story frequently to identify appearance beliefs or behaviors. Collect data on duration, intensity, and frequency of behaviors and thoughts. For example, if the patient reports that they engage in mirror checking as they brush their teeth, ask for details to elicit symptoms. How long did they get stuck inspecting, what were their thoughts as they inspected, how did they move on to the next task, and do triggers vary from day to day? Clinicians should document the day as a running list as illustrated below.

1. Patient woke at 9 a.m. Had the thought "I can't face another day. What if my hair looks worse?" As she walked toward the bathroom, were there more thoughts, mirrors in the hallways, etc.? What if they ran into a family member? (The idea here is to be very detail oriented).
2. Brushed teeth, tried not to look in mirror, and was able to walk away. Saw reflection in shower door that triggered mirror checking.
3. On the way to the kitchen for breakfast, walked past living room mirror. Lighting is always bad there. Saw hair as darker, making it look thicker. Had some hope that hair could look better today.

4. Showered. Hair not as thick after washing. Tried to style for 10 minutes. Mood more anxious.
5. Asked my mother if my hair looked good and she wouldn't answer. Thought "she sees it as worse."
6. Drove to work. Sat in parking lot inspecting hair in the car with rear-view mirror. Realized it was Tuesday, and staff meeting will be triggering due to close seating.

Functional Assessment of Compulsive Behaviors

> Collecting details of a typical day in the patient's life is a valuable tool to identify symptoms

A *functional assessment* is the cornerstone of CBT. It is a detailed understanding of the person's problematic thoughts and behaviors, along with the factors that influence their initiation and maintenance. A functional analysis is often referred to as an *ABC* model. The "A" stands for the antecedent triggers; both internal (cognitions and emotions) and external triggers (environmental events or circumstances). The "B" refers to the target behaviors, which are the compulsive and avoidance behaviors. The "C" refers to the consequences of the behavior, which include both the short-term and long-term cognitive, emotional, behavioral, and environmental outcomes of the behavior. For example, seeing oneself in the mirror may trigger sadness and an inspection of the "flaw." This may be followed by extensive mirror checking and excessive use of makeup to camouflage that "flaw." The consequence may be a decrease in anxiety and sadness in public (short term), but these behaviors are likely to lead to more mirror checking and camouflaging (long term). Discussion about the negative impact of avoidance and compulsive behaviors forms the basis for introducing later behavioral exercises in ERP (see Exposure and Response Prevention Therapy in Section 4.1.4: Cognitive Behavior Therapy for BDD).

Functional Assessment of Mirror Use

For BDD, a thorough functional analysis is helpful in understanding more prevalent and multifaceted daily behaviors, such as mirror checking or avoidance, skin picking, and grooming rituals. In particular, mirror checking can involve a complex set of antecedent triggers, followed by a sense of relief that maintains the behavior.

Cognitive triggers and consequences related to the mirror can consist of magical thinking. This may include beliefs such as: (1) my body part changes regularly, and I need to look to monitor the changes; (2) I need to achieve a good image of myself before I can leave the mirror; (3) I want to see myself like I did when I was younger (or more attractive, etc.). The intermittent reinforcement that mirror checking provides can maintain the behavior.

Identification of Etiological Environmental Variables

Life experiences may be important in the patient's own narrative and understanding of the etiology of their BDD. Individuals with BDD have histories with rates of physical, sexual, and emotional abuse greater than in the general population (Didie et al., 2006; Neziroglu et al., 2006) as well as childhood bullying and teasing (Neziroglu et al., 2018). In fact, research has shown that individuals with BDD place importance on their childhood teasing experiences as etiological factors (Weingarden et al., 2017), recalling appearance-related teasing as more traumatic and vivid than others (Buhlmann et al., 2011). The clinician should get a clear history of these factors and the importance the patient places on them (see Appendix 2).

BDD patients may note other difficult life experiences as contributing factors, including timing and experience of puberty, experience with sports and physical activities, accidents or medical conditions which altered appearance (rosacea, cystic acne, skin conditions, broken nose), and familial values of appearance (whether stated explicitly or implicitly). In addition, it is important to consider the patient's perception of trauma or abuse regardless of normative definitions.

The patient can develop their own list (perhaps chronologically) of etiological factors to better conceptualize the development of the disorder (see Appendix 3).

Assess for early life experiences and their impact on etiology

4.1.2 Psychoeducation

Psychoeducation for BDD includes establishing the CBT model with a description of the factors in the development and maintenance of the condition. Assessment and psychoeducation are critical to successful treatment and should not be rushed. These early sessions also provide opportunities for building a strong therapeutic alliance. Many BDD patients have suffered silently for many years, and the chance to delve into their struggles can be a relief. Clinicians should be cognizant in these early stages of the need not to rush into cognitive therapy (CT) when gathering a patient's beliefs. Maintaining a nonjudgmental and empathic stance is especially important, as BDD patients can be sensitive to perceived rejection or criticism. Early information and psychoeducation sessions should be used as opportunities to build hope and enthusiasm for treatment. At all times, the therapist's credibility is very important, and thus in both the psychoeducation and assessment phase the questions should be posed with a clear understanding of BDD. Minimizing the concern can lead to discontinuation (e.g., when the therapist says, "I am bald, and it doesn't bother me").

Psychoeducation of the BDD Model
Clinicians can refer back to Chapter 2 as a guide to explaining the biological, psychological, and environmental models in depth.
1. *Biological factors:* Provide patients with a basic understanding of the most up-to-date research regarding possible genetic predisposition, serotonin dysfunction, and the abnormalities in visual processing that can contribute to the development of BDD. The visual processing research helps patients understand why their perceptual experience may differ from others and encourages the use a medical conceptualization of their disorder rather than a problem of appearance.
2. *Psychological factors:* These include personality styles, core beliefs, such as perfectionism and reinforcement history. This section also includes reviewing the model of negative and positive reinforcement that maintains BDD beliefs and behaviors. This sets the stage for the CBT model.

3. *Environmental factors:* These include the larger sociocultural messages of attractiveness, personal family and friends' values, and life experiences such as bullying, teasing, and abuse. CBT strategies to address traumatic memories can be incorporated into the treatment protocol.

4.1.3 Treatment Orientation and Engagement

> **Patients should be informed of the collaborative nature of CBT**

Patients who have previously received general psychotherapy or have never sought therapy may not be prepared for the shift in the directive and structured style of CBT. Clinicians should orient patients regarding what to expect, and discuss their concerns. This is also a good opportunity to dispel any misconceptions about CBT. It is important to emphasize the collaborative nature of CBT, to ease fears about the treatment process, especially regarding ERP. Patients in CBT sometimes believe that the therapist's role is solely that of a "BDD therapist," and may not disclose other life issues. It is important to clarify your willingness to address all aspects of a person's life, stressors, and familial difficulties.

Goal Clarification: Body Image Versus Appearance

Successful treatment often starts with a shared conceptualization of the problem. Often the main obstacle in this population is disagreement regarding the diagnosis, resulting in difficulty arriving at an acceptable treatment goal. At this stage, clinicians should not attempt to engage in a direct debate, but rather indicate that there are two theories: *Theory A:* that there is a flaw in physical appearance that needs fixing, and *Theory B:* that there is a mental representation in the mind of a flaw in appearance, and the mental representation needs changing. Patients are told that Theory A is the one that they have held onto for a long time with no apparent change, and perhaps it is time to give Theory B a chance. Here the therapist tries to engage the patient to loosely commit to giving Theory B a chance at least for a few months. Clarify that appearance refers to the actual observable body parts, and body image is the picture we have of ourselves in our mind. Appearance does not change unless it is anatomically altered, whereas body image can be changed.

> **Distinguish appearance vs. body image to help develop a shared conceptualization**

Often the resulting compromise is an agreement to address the distress and functioning resulting from the preoccupation and to attack the mental representation of one's appearance. We advise clinicians to be flexible in these early discussions while still maintaining a firm stance that BDD is a problem of body image that is merely a mental representation of what we look like. A mental representation is composed of perceptions (sensory and visual input), emotions, and cognitions. Reviewing the definition of "body image" establishes the distinction between these two concepts. Something like this may be used to explain the definition of body image to the patient:

> None of us know how we look except by seeing a reflection of ourselves; most often in the mirror. We have a mental representation in our mind of the way we look, and this representation is composed of more than just the reflection in the mirror. It also includes our beliefs, our values, and our emotions. If we can change on or more aspects of this mental representation, we can change the way we feel about the way we look.

Motivational Interviewing

Motivational interviewing (MI; Miller & Rollnick, 1991, 2012) is a strategy initially designed to help individuals with addictions to commit to change. MI is a collaborative conversation style that encourages individuals to identify and resolve their own ambivalence regarding change. The patient is led by the clinician to articulate their own life goals and action plan for change. The following is a brief introduction to the basic principles and strategies of MI from Miller and Rollnick.

There are four key processes in MI. The first is *engaging*, which is establishing a strong therapeutic relationship by building mutual respect, expressing empathy, and focusing on the patient's strengths. The relationship is a collaborative partnership rather than a power dynamic between therapist and patient. The second key process, *focusing*, involves encouraging the person to identify what is truly important, identifying areas of "stuckness," and setting goals accordingly. *Evoking* is the third process, which refers to discovering the patient's own motivation to change. The clinician listens for statements that reflect an openness to change. The last step is *planning* for change. Patients may have a desire to change but not know how to start or engage in the process. Therapists should continue to empower the patient to create their own plan and refrain from taking over the planning stages unless requested to do so by the patient.

MI consists of four main communication skills abbreviated as OARS: *open-ended questions*, *affirming*, *reflective listening*, and *summarizing*. This style promotes a genuine nonjudgmental relationship between the patient and therapist. These techniques are woven into all conversations that occur in the course of MI. Some of the main principles of MI include expressing empathy, avoiding argument and confrontation, developing a discrepancy between the patient's behavior and their values and goals, rolling with resistance, maintaining optimism, and increasing patient's self-efficacy. An example of expressing empathy may be, "I can imagine how difficult it must be for you to feel so misunderstood by your mother about how you feel about your skin. No one seems to understand how you live day in and day out." Developing a discrepancy may look like this: "On the one hand you want to go back to school and socialize, but on the other hand, you feel too ugly to do so." Rolling with resistance occurs when the therapists says, "It is maybe too hard for you to come to therapy at this time. You don't seem to have a lot of time." You can instill self-efficacy by letting them know they have been able to deal with other painful situations in their life, they have been able to tolerate anxiety in the past, and they can do it now as well.

When conducting MI for BDD, it is important to acknowledge the patient's perspective on *both* the benefits and costs of the appearance preoccupation and perceived benefits of looking better. The patient can hopefully move forward by recognizing that the costs to their well-being, daily functioning, and suffering are far greater than the importance placed on appearance. A strong familiarity with and proficiency in MI are highly recommended for clinicians treating BDD. MI strategies are woven into many stages of the treatment whenever resistance or stagnation occurs – not merely at the beginning of treatment. Engagement in BDD treatment waxes and wanes throughout the treatment, requiring MI techniques to be regularly implemented.

Motivational interviewing is often necessary to engage patients in treatment

4.1.4 Cognitive Therapy

CBT consists of a multitude of techniques supported by a theoretical framework and research evidence. The focus of the treatment is on how current thoughts, behaviors, and emotions maintain the disorder. Interventions are based on identifying the dysfunctional beliefs and behaviors, and systematically altering those these patterns.

In a majority of cases, BDD treatment should start with MI and CT before implementing ERP.

Cognitive Therapy
Traditional *cognitive therapy* (CT) can be implemented in BDD with a careful approach, especially in those with high overvalued ideation or delusional thoughts. Individuals with BDD are sensitive and hypervigilant to any feedback on their appearance and can easily misinterpret examples or discussions about the existence of the perceived flaw. Therapists, therefore, have to be equally vigilant regarding possible areas of misunderstanding. For those with high overvalued ideation, targeting some of the less rigid beliefs first may lead to success; these often include beliefs about others' views of them. Challenging the patient's own views of themselves is often more difficult and requires a stronger therapeutic relationship.

The main focus of CT is to challenge core beliefs about self-worth, inadequacy, value on appearance, and the negative impact of the preoccupation on functioning and life goals. Other than these guidelines, CT in BDD can be applied using established protocols.

What To Say and Not To Say in Cognitive Therapy
Here are some specific suggestions on the types of conversations that should be avoided in the course of CT:

1. Do not dispute the existence of flaws; rather focus on the distress and overfocus on appearance and value. Acknowledge that there is a discrepancy between your perspective and their perspective regarding appearance.
2. Do not indicate that you see the flaw or state that it "isn't too bad" or "maybe it's a little noticeable only if you look closely."
3. Do not engage in reassurance either directly or indirectly that your patient looks attractive or normal. This may lead to the patient seeking reassurance from you in the future. It also gives the message that one person's opinion is important or accurate. Instead engage the patient in a discussion of decreasing their reliance on others' opinions.
4. Be cautious in discussing the concept of "worst case scenario" regarding the existence of a flaw, especially in the early stages of CT. Accepting a worst case is often misinterpreted by the patient to mean you see their flaw too, even if it is posed as a hypothetical scenario. A BDD patient may be devastated by even entertaining that possibility and may fixate on it throughout the course of treatment. Discussing the worst case of not being the most-sought-after person at a party or being judged critically by others can be a productive conversation. In later sessions, once the patient is more schooled in CT, it is possible to entertain the worst

case of the existence of appearance flaws, depending on the degree of overvalued ideation. Assessing overvalued ideation as CT progresses may provide a benchmark for treatment planning.

As in standard CT protocols, patients should record their automatic thoughts in a thought record and be guided to identify cognitive distortions. Cognitive distortions are the patterns of unhelpful cognitive errors or biases in thinking. As patients record their automatic thoughts multiple times, these distortions become more evident. Appendix 4 provides some examples of BDD-related cognitive distortions.

Levels of Beliefs in Cognitive Therapy

CT can be thought of concentric circles with automatic thoughts on the surface, followed by intermediate beliefs, and core beliefs in the center. To achieve the best chance of long-term cognitive shift toward balanced thinking, it is recommended that clinicians identify, challenge, and replace unhealthy intermediate and core beliefs. Intermediate beliefs are defined as rules and assumptions that apply across situations. Core beliefs are defined by Beck (1976) as "deeply held beliefs about self, others, and the world." Automatic thoughts are the surface level thoughts that get activated in day-to-day life situations.

Examples of Automatic Thoughts
"My nose is big."
"I have a lot of pimples."

Examples of Intermediate Beliefs
"If my appearance is flawed, then I am flawed."
"If I am unattractive, then life is not worth living."
"The more attractive you are, the better your life."
"Attractive people get ahead in life."
"I will not get a partner, because of the way I look."
"Life is not worth living if I can't get surgery."
"One of the most important things in life is attractiveness."
"To keep your partner, you should always stay youthful and attractive."
"I would give a million dollars not to have that flaw."
"If I'm muscular, then people will love me."
"People with good skin are happier and have a better life."

Examples of Core Beliefs

About Self	*About Others*	*About the World*
"I'm inadequate."	"Others can't be trusted."	"The world is a dangerous place."
"I'm unlovable."	"People are out to get me."	
"I'm worthless."		
"I'm abnormal."		

Challenging Intermediate and Core Beliefs

Identifying core beliefs can be done in a few different ways. Clinicians and patients can review completed automatic thought records to identify patterns and clues about deeper beliefs. Another common method is called the *downward arrow technique* in which the clinician asks the patient questions about an automatic thought, until the core belief is uncovered. Common questions include "what does that thought mean?" and "if that were true, then what?" Continue the questioning until the patient is unable to identify a deeper belief. Typically core beliefs in BDD regard self-worth and inadequacy. Appendix 5 is a thought record homework sheet for patients to use.

Challenging the Value of Appearance

Values are defined as principles that guide our choices and include our moral sense of right and wrong, our priorities, and ideas that matter in our life. They are the compass by which we live, guiding how we behave and who we want to be. Values are not static; they are evaluated and pursued throughout life. However, people often mistake goals and values. Goals are more specific, desired objectives or benchmarks to achieve. For example, living a healthy lifestyle is a *value* whereas exercising three times a week is a *goal*. Values help us create goals to work toward. ACT includes helpful values clarification. Appendix 6 is a worksheet exercise on values clarification and the discrepancy between desired values and the actual time spent on these values in one's life.

Discrepancy in Values Exercise

1. Have your patient make a list of all of their life values. It may be helpful to provide a list of values to use as a reference. Allow them to include appearance if they choose.
2. Ask your patient to decide the importance of each value by assigning it a percentage out of a 100. The total sum should not be more than 100.
3. Next, diagram the values on a pie chart and label it "Desired Values."
4. Ask them to identify how much time they actually devote to each of their values during the week.
5. Draw a second pie chart diagram and label it "Time Spent on Values."

The goal of the exercise is to identify the discrepancy between articulated values and the time and importance given to a select few (e.g., appearance and being accepted by others). Engage the patient in a discussion regarding the obstacles to living by one's values. For example, perhaps they identify education as a value, but their fear of being judged for the size of their nose interferes with behaviors that support that value by attending school. How much time do they spend on their education (5% of their day) versus the importance they rated it (20%)?

Examples of values: achievement, autonomy, adventure, appearance, excitement, fame, faith, family, friendship, health, helpfulness, humor, loyalty, power, spirituality, stability, and wealth.

4.1.5 Exposure and Response Prevention

ERP in BDD is best implemented gradually

Exposure and response prevention (ERP) is a scientifically supported treatment that helps patients face (exposure) their feared and avoided triggers (situations, thoughts, images, objects) while eliminating compulsive behaviors. ERP is an opportunity to challenge beliefs by confronting situations in which they can be experienced and tested. New learning takes place when predicted outcomes do not occur. Patients learn that they can habituate or learn to tolerate their discomfort. In the case of BDD, triggers may include well-lit crowded social situations, photographs of themselves, viewing attractive celebrities, and having mental images of themselves at a younger age. In ERP, the therapist asks the patient to engage in response prevention (not to check mirrors or avoid them, and no camouflaging, no grooming rituals, no reassurance seeking, etc.) in the face of these triggers. ERP is conducted in a gradual manner and at a pace the patient is able to tolerate.

ERP for BDD, although guided by successful treatment for OCD, cannot typically be implemented at the same pace or intensity. BDD patients may experience an increase in shame, depression, and suicidal thoughts, especially if overvalued ideation is high. It is strongly advised that the decision to institute ERP is guided by an assessment of the patient's proficiency in CT, their suicide risk, and their general emotion regulation skills. It is also beneficial if the patient has begun to decrease compulsive mirror checking routines or self-examination, so they do not deteriorate subsequent to exposure exercises.

In Vivo Versus Imaginal Exposures

ERP can be conducted in vivo and/or in the patient's imagination. In vivo exposures are conducted in the natural environment whereas imaginal exposures consist of imagery and scripts of feared scenarios. In vivo exercises provide opportunities to fully immerse patients in real situations. Imaginal exercises may be helpful in certain circumstances – for example, when a situation is not possible to create in real life or when the patient is too fearful of or resistant to in vivo exercises. The combination of both modalities may lead to more lasting gains. Flooding a patient by articulating their fears during in vivo exposures is an effective approach in OCD, whereas in BDD, it should be very gradually introduced when used with in vivo exposures. Use of humor during flooding can be used more freely in OCD, but should again be used minimally or with extreme caution during BDD exposure treatment.

Therapist-Guided Versus Self-Guided Exposure Therapy

We strongly advise therapists to conduct exposure exercises during sessions rather than relying on homework compliance alone. The benefit of therapist-guided exposures is that it ensures compliance. It also allows the therapist to monitor a patient's subtle avoidance, engagement in self-reassurance, or engaging in other behaviors that are counter-therapeutic. Treatment gains and adherence are higher with therapist-guided exposure within the OCD literature (Tolin et al., 2007).

In-session ERP facilitates treatment adherence

Preparing the Patient

Exposure exercises in BDD can illicit numerous painful emotions in addition to anxiety, such as shame, disgust, depression, and hopelessness. Clinicians should thoroughly assess whether their patient understands the rationale behind ERP and is prepared for the challenging experiences. A collaborative approach is the key, with the understanding that the patient is has an integral part to play in deciding the pace and intensity of the exercises.

Early exposure exercises can be framed as collaborative empirical experiments to gather data on the validity of their beliefs. For example, "Do other people really treat me differently with and without my camouflage makeup or a hat?" "Do others notice my skin blemishes as I predict?" and "Can I tolerate exposing my perceived defect in public?"

In moderate-to-severe BDD, initial exposures may consist of simple trips to public places. For patients who have been largely housebound or have had very limited daily activity, trips out of the therapy office may serve as behavioral activation or simply to help them engage in the world again. In these cases, clinicians should refrain from increasing the difficulty of the exposures, but should instead focus on improving quality of life by helping patients go to places they may have avoided. We encourage you to maximize reinforcement and strongly encourage patients' progress in leaving their homes.

Later exercises can include avoided situations and scenarios in which the body part is deliberately more visible or pronounced. Clinicians should proceed cautiously throughout ERP for BDD. ERP may occasionally need to be halted to address an increase in depression or suicidality. Flexibility is required in pacing, and at times, resuming earlier exposures may be necessary. You may need to reengage the patient in treatment at times.

Response Reduction and Prevention

Reducing safety-seeking behaviors and mirror checking, before implementing exposure exercises can be early opportunities to implement behavioral change. Patients are often willing to decrease mirror checking early on in the therapeutic process, as opposed to decreasing other behaviors, such as social avoidance or camouflaging. Reducing mirror checking allows the patient to better manage their emotional distress after exposure exercises, so special attention should be given to helping the patient reduce that mirror checking.

Reducing mirror checking is difficult for patients, and extra support is necessary

We are often asked if the treatment plan is to never look in a mirror again. In fact, eliminating mirrors and reflective surfaces is not possible or practical. For this reason, the goal of response prevention is to eliminate the compulsive use of the mirror and learn to use mirrors for a functional reason. When patients are struggling significantly with reducing urges to mirror check, it is helpful to temporarily cover some mirrors and remove others from the home. However, the long-term goal is to have existing mirrors remain in place while the patient learns to use mirrors as others do. We encourage patients to use the mirror to shave, put makeup on, blow-dry their hair, brush their teeth, wash their face, or to look at themselves globally in a full-length mirror before they go out. All nonessential mirror usage is discouraged.

Clinicians should develop a structured plan to reduce and eliminate all other compulsive behaviors systematically in conjunction with exposure exercises once the patient has self-monitored and created a list of all of these behaviors (see Appendix 7).

Developing a Hierarchy

A hierarchy is a ranked list of all the external and internal triggers that cause distress, as well as of avoided situations. The hierarchy is symptom specific to each body part, although overlap can exist. Numerical ratings are assigned to the items on the list, often called a *subjective units of distress* (SUDs). A scale of 1 to 10, or 10 to a 100, can be used, with lower items indicating less distress. Patients can either choose which body part to target, based on which is less anxiety provoking or which causes the most daily functional impairment and distress. A review of the typical day can assist in constructing a hierarchy since it highlights areas of difficulty (see Appendix 8).

Sample Exposure Hierarchy: Facial Skin Redness
100 Hot sunny day at a crowded park
100 Going to the beach
 90 Doing a group exercise class
 80 Posting photos of oneself on social media
 80 Exercise at a gym when not crowded
 70 Going shopping without makeup
 70 Taking a walk outdoors on a sunny day
 60 Eating spicy food at a restaurant
 65 Wearing a red shirt and other colors that accentuate skin redness
 50 Shopping for clothes and use of dressing rooms
 40 Interacting with strangers briefly
 30 Seeing family members, without having makeup on

Conducting Exposure In-Session

Conducting successful exposure therapy relies on careful collaborative planning before each exercise. Clarify what symptom and belief is being targeted during that session, agree upon a real-life or imaginal experience, agree on response prevention following the exposure, and discuss the patient's reaction afterwards. For example, if you are targeting a patient's avoidance and distress shopping for clothes, you may be targeting the following beliefs: (1) "Others will notice and judge me negatively"; (2) "I won't find anything that fits me."

A longer session of a minimum of 90 minutes is recommended to conduct the exposure and have adequate time to discuss the patient's reaction after the exercise. Usually, the sessions are longer in duration and more frequent during the initial stages of treatment.

Once an item on the hierarchy is chosen and planned, the patient and therapist can engage in the exercise. Creating scenarios to address hierarchy items requires creativity and advance planning. Therapists should be familiar with public areas near their office that offer a variety of experiences, such as lighting variations, number of mirrors, level of crowds, opportunities to interact with strangers, local gyms that offer free trial memberships, etc.

During the experience, the therapist should prompt the patient to rate their SUDs level a few times. It may be helpful to record these numbers to demonstrate that distress reduction does occur during exposures and with repetitions of the same exposure. At times, SUDs levels do not decrease appreciably during the exposure. This is not necessarily a cause for concern. Identify whether that experience requires additional practice, if the difficulty level needs to be adjusted for the next session, or if the patient was triggered by other factors. For example, if a department store with many mirrors led to mirror checking and increased distress, then future exposures can be planned in a different location.

Plan for longer sessions when incorporating ERP

Clinicians are often uncomfortable being in a public place with a patient and may therefore rush through the exercises. Successful exposures require some patience and sufficient time spent in an anxiety-provoking situation. Clinicians should work toward presenting a relaxed and natural demeanor.

It is also worth preplanning how you will protect the patient's confidentiality should you run into an acquaintance, or if a stranger asks about your relationship.

Debriefing

Debriefing consolidates learning during ERP

Debriefing after an exposure is critical to assess whether the intended cognitive shift matched the patient's perspective on their experience. Asking the patient what they learned during the exercise helps identify and clarify any misinterpretations and consolidates learning. It also identifies ongoing cognitive distortions and automatic thoughts, which can be challenged before the session ends. Ask the patient to assess whether their predicted and actual experience matched. Were they accurate in the level of distress they predicted? What did they learn from the experience?

Debriefing should also include a review of the agreed-upon response prevention that will occur after session and before the next appointment. Engage in MI, CT, or problem solving to help the patient adhere to the response prevention plan.

Planning Homework

Behavior therapy relies on the process of generalization of treatment gains *during* and *between* sessions. To facilitate learning, patients should be encouraged to engage in structured homework assignments. It is advisable to assign homework assignments that are a repetition of the ones already practiced in session. Patients typically struggle with increased distress when practicing independently versus practicing with the support of their therapist. For this reason, assigning homework that is too challenging can decrease treatment adherence. Assign homework that is somewhat easier than the patient can handle in the early stages of treatment. For imaginal exposures, the patient should have a copy of the script to read daily or an audio recording to listen to. Homework compliance leads to more positive treatment outcomes in psychotherapy (Mausbach et al., 2010).

Home Visits

Home visits are helpful to address grooming or mirror-checking routines that impact patient's ability to leave home. In severe cases, individuals with BDD are homebound and refuse to be seen by others. In this case, home visits may be the only opportunity for a patient to receive treatment. Not all clinicians are able to accommodate home visits, but when possible, these sessions can provide valuable information on a patient's daily routines. Teletherapy can also be implemented with use of video sessions as a substitute for in-person home visits. Coaching a patient to decrease their morning grooming routine, as they are engaging in it, may lead to quicker progress in reducing and eliminating these behaviors.

Should the Mirror Be Used as an Exposure Exercise?

Mirror exposures are usually discouraged during the course of treatment. Mirror use during a session typically results in compulsive checking and reassurance seeking, causing an increase in the patient's distress rather than a reduction in symptoms.

Mirror use during a session may be warranted in the following circumstances: (1) for patients who engage in significant mirror avoidance, (2) to practice resisting the urge to check, and (3) for mirror retraining as described in the next section.

4.1.6 Perceptual Retraining

Patients rely heavily on their visual experience in assessing their appearance. Despite psychoeducation regarding visual processing distortions evident in BDD, patients understandably have significant difficulty dismissing their own sensory input and may repeatedly express the claim that they "see the defect," despite understanding the concept of detail versus holistic processing. In-session exercises to demonstrate this perceptual phenomenon can be a valuable tool to strengthen the patient's understanding.

Perceptual retraining illustrates detail vs. holistic visual processing

Holistic Perceptual Training
The following exercises may be beneficial in demonstrating and teaching the patient how detail versus holistic processing impacts the development and/or maintenance of their disorder and how emotions can impact their experience. It is recommended that this exercise be repeated and implemented before mirror retraining. Learning holistic processing with neutral images may facilitate the acquisition of holistic processing of one's own image (see Appendix 9).

Holistic Perceptual Training Exercise 1
The goal of this exercise is to demonstrate how detail focus alters one's perceptual experience of visual stimuli.
 1. Choose detailed photographs or images unfamiliar to the patient, such as a full bookcase, a painting, a landscape photograph, or an image of an object similar in detail.
 2. Ask the patient to list all of the things they notice in the image. Encourage them to list objects, size, shape, and colors present in the image.
 3. Ask the patient to rate the image on a scale of 1 to 10, with 1 being unpleasant or unattractive, 5 being neutral, and 10 being very pleasant.
 4. Instruct the patient to focus on one particular aspect of the image – for example, a particular book, a branch of a tree, or a small detail in the painting such as the hand of a person in a portrait.
 5. Ask the patient to stare at that one small area for a full minute.
 6. Take the image away for a period and do not discuss it further. Perhaps review therapy homework during that time in-session.
 7. Reintroduce the same image 15 minutes later. What do they notice now? What aspect of the image first drew their visual attention? Was it the area they had been instructed to stare at before? How did their experience of the image change after focusing on the detail? In other words, did they experience the image as pleasant, neutral, or unpleasant? Use the scale of 1–10 as you did initially.
 8. Repeat with multiple images over a couple of sessions.

9. Tie in this exercise to their perception in the mirror (how does repeated examination and focus on details alter their overall opinion and experience of an image?).
10. Reinforce psychoeducation of visual processing in BDD.

Holistic Perceptual Training Exercise 2

Exercise 1 can be repeated in a somewhat different form by choosing a couple of images with actual slight imperfections, such as a crooked book, imperfect brush stroke, or dead leaf on a tree.

1. Ask the patient to first look at the full image and rate their opinion of it on a scale of 1 to 10, with 1 being an unpleasant image, 5 being neutral, and 10 being a very pleasant image.
2. Now draw their attention to the slight imperfection and ask them to stare at it for a minute.
3. Take the image away and move on to other agenda items in-session. Do not discuss the image.
4. Reintroduce the same image 15 minutes later. What do they notice now? What aspect of the image first drew their visual attention? Was it the area they had been instructed to stare at before? How did their experience of the image change after focusing on the detail?
5. Repeat with multiple images over a couple of sessions.
6. Reflect on how focusing on certain areas of a visual image alters one's overall opinion of it.

Impact of Emotions and Cognitions on Visual Perception

Neurologists have long recognized that our senses elicit emotional, cognitive, behavioral, and physiological experiences. For example, smelling warm chocolate chip cookies activates certain pleasant memories and emotions, whereas a horror movie can activate less pleasant cognitions and emotions. But the reverse connection, that our emotions alter our perception, is still under debate (Niedenthal & Wood, 2019). Some preliminary neuroimaging research in BDD suggests that emotional arousal is associated with less activity in the dorsal visual stream, which is a brain region responsible for holistic processing (Feusner, Moody, et al., 2010), indicating that there is a possible influence of emotions on visual perception of one's face. Perhaps further research will clarify this concept.

Most individuals with BDD will acknowledge that their expectations, emotional state, and cognitions *before* they approach the mirror influence how they judge themselves in the mirror. Whether this is the result of an actual bidirectional relationship between neuroanatomical circuitry and emotions is yet to be proven. Experientially we know that if you feel happy you are more likely to think you are more attractive, be friendlier, and see the world in a more positive light than if you are depressed. We label someone as depressed if we observe they have a slouched back, slower movements, slower speech, and lower voice tone accompanied by a dislike of themselves and their appearance. This indicates a correlation between emotions, gestures, movements, and self-perception. Because there seems to be a relationship between emotions and interpretation of visual input, it is helpful to teach patients to identify and challenge their beliefs before they approach the mirror, and practice CT skills before they look at themselves.

Mirror Retraining

Mirror retraining is a treatment technique developed by Wilhelm and colleagues to help patients learn holistic versus detailed processing of appearance and to learn to use nonjudgmental language regarding one's appearance (Wilhelm et al., 2013) and is incorporated regularly in BDD treatment.

Mirror retraining involves looking at oneself in the mirror and describing one's appearance in objective language. Wilhelm and colleagues suggest the following guidance on conducting mirror retraining (Wilhelm et al., 2012). Patients can create a hierarchy of the type and size of mirrors, the distance from the mirror, angle, and lighting, and choose the easiest type of mirror to practice the exercise. The clinician should first demonstrate and model the exercise. Starting at the top of the head and working down to the feet, describe the size, shape, and color of body parts in a neutral way. For example, "My hair is shoulder length, dark brown with some red highlights, my eyes are round, my nose is about two inches long," and so on. Clinicians should elicit a rating of anxiety to assess the patient's experience. For some patients, small mirrors or dark lighting may be the only way they can tolerate this exercise. The ultimate goal is to use a full-length mirror so the patient can engage in holistic visual processing. Clinicians can coach and correct any judgmental language used by the patient. The exercise should be repeated and practiced as homework.

> Mirror retraining teaches holistic processing and nonjudgmental language about one's appearance

4.2 Mechanisms of Action

A diathesis–stress model suggests that BDD etiology can be explained by an interaction between neurobiological predisposition and environmental influences such as social learning and conditioning events. Evaluative conditioning is theorized to explain both symptom acquisition and maintenance of BDD-specific behaviors. Evaluative conditioning is similar to classical conditioning, with the latter referring to physiological responses, and the former to attitudes toward, or likes and dislikes of the conditioned stimuli. The negative evaluations are maintained via avoidance behaviors, which become negatively reinforcing by the elimination of unpleasant negative experiences. For example, early negative experiences, such as teasing, acne, abuse, difficult puberty, or physical injury (unconditioned stimuli) result in a negative emotional response (unconditioned emotional response), such as anxiety, disgust, shame, and sadness. Stimuli that are paired with those negative experiences (conditioned stimuli) result in the same negative reactions (conditioned emotional responses). These conditioned stimuli involve body parts and aspects of appearance as well as certain words via relational frame theory (red, skin, small). Avoidance of situations that trigger these negative emotions becomes reinforcing.

ERP is based on the model of fear extinction by repeated exposure and experience to the conditioned stimuli without the avoidance or compensatory behaviors to reduce anxiety. Until recently, it was believed that habituation, or reducing anxiety, was necessary for effective exposure therapy. But, although habituation can and does occur in many clinical situations, it does not always

> Evaluative conditioning may explain the acquisition and maintenance of symptoms

do so. Furthermore, positive treatment outcomes can occur with *or* without habituation.

More recently, the inhibitory learning theory of Craske and colleagues more accurately demonstrates the mechanism of action for ERP, by suggesting that the original fear associations do not disappear or become unlearned (Craske et al., 2014). The old learning stays intact and is instead replaced with newer safety information. For exposure therapy to result in maximum gains and "inhibit" the old learning, it should be conducted across a variety of situations, be designed to disconfirm predictions with carefully targeted exercises, and create an element of surprise (i.e., exposure exercises that are not always preplanned in detail and which increase the intensity of the exercise).

CT aims to challenge and replace core maladaptive beliefs, resulting in a decrease in negative emotions and resulting BDD behaviors. It also aims to reduce self-focused attention and biases in information processing that influence the acquisition and maintenance of BDD beliefs.

> **Inhibitory learning theory explains the mechanism of ERP**

4.3 Efficacy and Prognosis

Research outcomes for studies of CBT for BDD are promising, as measured by a handful of randomized trials comparing CBT to waitlist controls. When compared with anxiety management, CBT is more effective (Veale et al., 2014). CBT has been efficacious for delusional BDD, with insight improving post-treatment. Treatment has been shown to be helpful using individual (McKay et al., 1997; McKay, 1999) and group formats (Wilhelm et al., 1999), and with Internet-delivered modalities (Enander et al., 2016). The research has demonstrated that response rates vary from 48% to 82% in measurable improvement. Randomized clinical trials have shown positive treatment outcomes (Rosen et al., 1995; Veale et al., 1996; Wilhelm et al., 2014), as have numerous studies and case series with smaller sample sizes. Treatment outcome has been shown to be predicted by readiness or motivation for change, treatment expectancy, and insight. Addressing quality of life and developing a thorough relapse prevention plan can ensure long-term treatment gains.

> **CBT response rates are 48% to 82% in measurable improvement**

The course of BDD is chronic, and lack of treatment response is predicted by more severe symptoms at intake, longer duration of BDD, being an adult, and the presence of comorbid personality disorder (Phillips et al., 2013; Phillips, Pagano et al., 2006, 2013). Left untreated, BDD is unlikely to spontaneously improve (Phillips et al., 2006, 2013).

4.4 Variations and Combinations of Methods

The severity and presentation of BDD should inform the treatment plan. CBT and ERP alone may not be sufficient to achieve clinically significant change. Session frequency and length may need to be adjusted to match your patient's impairment level. CT as described above should typically precede ERP treatment. Even if the patient reports previous CT with another clini-

> **Medications are often a necessary component of successful treatment**

cian, repetition of the treatment as well as a specialized approach is strongly recommended.

ERP for BDD is likely to be most effective when conducted gradually, when it is therapist guided, and when it incorporates sufficient time for debriefing to address the patient's perception of the experience. ERP in a real public environment can result in misperceptions based on selective attention to certain variables over others. Clinicians should pay careful attention to their patient's mood and reaction, to correct possible inaccurate conclusions.

Adding medication to psychological treatment is standard in most clinical settings, although there is insufficient research to make definitive conclusions as to whether the addition of medication improves treatment outcomes. Given the rigorous outcome research in OCD and research documenting the high risk in BDD, it is fair to conclude that medications are often a necessary component of a successful outcome. BDD typically responds best to higher doses of SSRIs than are typically used in depression (Phillips, 2010).

4.4.1 Attentional Training Technique and Task Concentration

The *attentional training technique* (ATT; Wells, 1990) is a metacognitive therapy that develops a person's ability to switch attention away from nonrelevant or internal experiences toward more relevant stimuli. The goal is to (1) reduce self-focused attention and (2) increase attentional control and flexibility. ATT has been implemented for social phobia with success (Clark & Wells, 1995), lending itself to viable treatment for BDD.

Task concentration training (TCT; Bogels, 2006) involves developing an ability to focus attention away from internal experiences, such as one's thoughts, to the immediate environment or tasks one is engaged in. The goal is to demonstrate the negative impact of internal focus on maintaining preoccupation and distress and interfering with the ability to engage in activities or relate to others. ATT and TCT have some similarities to mindfulness, in which the goal is to disengage from internal judgments and experiences toward the present moment.

> ATT and TCT teach patients to switch focus from internal experiences to externally relevant tasks and stimuli

Individuals with BDD typically display two biases in their attention and focus (Veale & Neziroglu, 2010); the first is hypervigilance to specific aspects of a stimuli or situation, and the second is internal focus on one's own thoughts, emotions, and behaviors. In the first bias, for example, the person may only notice attractive people and the fun they are having, and in the second bias, the person pays attention to how unattractive they are compared with others, believing that if only they looked better they would have more people talking to them. These attentional biases confirm their preconceived beliefs and lead to missing relevant information that might provide an alternate perspective. For example, if a person believes that everyone with good facial features is happy, they may scan a room full of people at a party for attractive people who seem happy without noticing all the other guests displaying a variety of other emotions.

ATT and TCT can be taught with self-monitoring and in-session exercises, followed by homework exercises to practice decreasing internal focus; widening one's attention in a situation; and increasing focusing on, and switching between, internal and external focus to strengthen attentional flexibility.

The following are some exercises to teach ATT and TCT (Veale & Neziroglu, 2010).

Before you start the exercise, first assess your patient's level of internal or external focus. Ask the patient to rate themselves from –3 (totally internally focused) to +3 (totally externally focused) with 0 being equally internally and externally focused. Most individuals with BDD rate themselves as –2 or –3. As you go through these exercises, and from session to session, have the patient rate their level of internal focus. You can also ask the patient to rate the percentage of focus on self, environment, and task. Most people who are not self-focused are usually 70% focused on the task, 10% on environmental sounds, and 20% on the self. Individuals with BDD are 80% or so focused on self. The following exercises are intended over time to increase task focus.

Task Concentration Training
Listening Exercise for TCT

Exercise 1: The patient and therapist sit with their backs to each other. The clinician tells a neutral 2-minute story, and the patient is told to pay attention and summarize as much of the story as they can. The patient is asked to rate the percentage of their attention on the task, self, and the environment. The patient and therapist rate how much of the story is recalled.

Exercise 2: The patient and therapist sit facing each other and make eye contact while the therapist tells another 2-minute neutral story. Again, the patient rates attention and percentage of story recall.

Exercise 3: The patient is told to become distracted by creating distress about their body part by possibly touching their body part twice or looking in a mirror placed near them. The patient listens to the therapist tell a neutral story and then tries to summarize the story paying attention to whether they lost parts of the story while they were self-focused after producing distress. This exercise is repeated until their focus on the task is above 50%.

Exercise 4: The therapist tells an appearance-related story for 2 minutes, and the patient is asked to summarize it again.

Speaking Exercises for TCT

These exercises are the same as above except the patient tells the story for 2 minutes under the same four scenarios, and pays attention to whether the therapist is listening and to what they are saying.

Task Concentration Exercise in Nonthreatening Situation

Have patient walk in a park, or cook meal, or engage in some other a nonthreatening task, while paying attention to the various sounds and colors.

Task Concentration Exercise in a Threatening Situation

Have the patient engage in a task that is distress producing, while concentrating on sounds, colors, forms, etc. in the environment. Each exercise should be practiced in-session and between sessions until the patient is able to concentrate on the task more than 50% of the time.

Attentional Training

Attentional training is designed to increase the patient's flexibility to switch their attention from internal to external focus at any time. It is to be practiced when not distressed so that a habit is formed and the patient can switch their focus when needed.

Switching Attention to Sounds

These exercises practice flexibility in attention and increasing focus on the environment.

Exercise 1: Gather about 6 to 8 sounds of different varieties. Some of these can be prerecorded or found on the Internet (e.g., instrumental music, wind chimes), some created in-session (sound of your voice or of tapping), and some can be found in the immediate environment (a fan or traffic sounds). The patient is asked to keep their eyes open and not suppress any thoughts or emotions, but to simply focus on the task. Create all of the sounds in the room at once. Guide the patient through focusing on one sound at a time, as you call it out. Pause at each sound. Shift their attention to sound 2 only, sound 3 only, and so on, until they are familiar with all of the sounds.

Exercise 2: Next, practice shifting quickly between the sounds in a random order as you call out the sound. Again, the patient is instructed to focus only on the sound you mention. Pause for a couple of seconds before moving to another sound.

Exercise 3: Finally, ask the patient to broaden their attention to all of the sounds at once.

Flexibility in switching attention outward can be done by training on sounds, colors, textures, and objects.

4.4.2 Cognitive Remediation

Cognitive remediation therapy (CRT) is a type of intensive therapy administered to individuals with psychiatric disorders involving symptomatic active neuropsychological deficits (Ikebuchi et al., 2017). Originally, cognitive remediation was used to aid patients suffering from brain lesions (Dahlgren et al., 2014), but more recently, it has been able to help individuals with psychiatric disorders as well. Because of its impact on executive functioning abilities, CRT has recently been used as a treatment for anorexia nervosa (AN).

Impairments associated with AN manifest themselves through self-imposed repetitive action and rules that involve excessively fixating on details to the detriment of global features (Tchanturia et al., 2012). BDD is often associated with similar impairments in executive functioning (Buhlmann & Wilhelm, 2004; Feusner, Neziroglu, et al., 2010; Greenberg et al., 2018). Both BDD and AN are rooted in rigid, repetitive, and harmful behaviors and thought processes that result in deficits in executive functioning, cognition, and global perception (Savage et al., 1999). In CRT, several activities and exercises are carried out to "exercise" different neural circuits that may be experiencing deficits (Vita et al., 2016). The exercises are designed to produce an indirect effect and improve overall functioning and quality of life. These processes can include attention, memory, executive function, social cognition, improvement of dysfunctional thinking styles, or metacognition (van Passel et al., 2016). A preliminary study using CRT as an adjunct to ERP shows promise in improving BDD symptoms (T. Borda and F. Neziroglu, personal communication, July 20, 2017).

4.4.3 Third Wave Therapies

The following third wave approaches are recommended when standard CBT for BDD is difficult for the patient to engage in, due to continued low motivation, suicidal ideation, emotion dysregulation, or persistent high overvalued ideation despite CT, or if the patient has difficulty tolerating the discomfort or distress of ERP.

Dialectical Behavior Therapy
Dialectical behavior therapy (DBT) was initially developed by Marsha Linehan (1993) to address chronic suicidality and self-injury in adolescents. It is an empirically validated treatment for borderline personality disorders. DBT incorporates CBT theory with Eastern beliefs of acceptance in order to balance change and validation interventions. The treatment module consists of individual therapy, skills training typically in a group format, therapist consultation, and telephone coaching for patients. The skills taught in DBT consist of mindfulness, emotion regulation, distress tolerance, and interpersonal effectiveness.

Many of the skills taught in DBT are helpful for patients with BDD and can be incorporated to build coping skills. Patients can benefit from the structured way that mindfulness skills are taught in DBT with daily practice and worksheets. The distress tolerance skills, which include self-soothing, distraction, and improving the moment, are helpful for patients who become easily emotionally dysregulated or have little control over their urges to mirror check or skin pick.

DBT should be strongly considered when the patient's symptoms of borderline personality disorder are interfering with the ability to engage in BDD treatment. In some cases, the personality disorder may need to be addressed prior to, or in conjunction with, BDD treatment. Chronic suicidality can also be effectively addressed with DBT.

Acceptance and Commitment Therapy
Acceptance and commitment therapy (ACT; Hayes, Strosahl, & Wilson, 2011) is an empirically validated treatment that aims to teach psychological flexibility with mindfulness practice, which can result in meaningful behavior change. ACT has six core processes: (1) cognitive defusion, (2) acceptance, (3) connection with present moment, (4) observing self, (5) values clarification, and (6) committed action. ACT uses metaphors, paradox, and exercises to teach these skills. For BDD patients, ACT can be used as an adjunct to CBT to increase treatment engagement, develop skills for responding to beliefs that are overvalued, increase willingness to tolerate unpleasant experiences, and engender a commitment to engaging in life. ACT's emphasis on living a valued life despite one's symptoms may also be particularly applicable to BDD to target quality of life. Some preliminary research supports the use of

acceptance-based strategies for BDD (Dehbaneh, 2019; Linde et al., 2015). Three of the six processes of ACT will be illustrated below as they can be applied to BDD.

Application of ACT to BDD

Cognitive defusion aims to teach that thoughts are simply internal events that do not have to be attended to, obeyed, or believed. Thoughts are not necessarily a reflection of reality. Cognitive defusion exercises are designed to teach ways to step back from thoughts and be less dictated to by rigid judgments. If CT strategies are not sufficient to decrease the strength of the appearance beliefs, cognitive defusion may help patients decrease their engagement in the thoughts. Defusing from thoughts can lessen their impact on behaviors.

In one exercise, the patient is encouraged to:
1. Treat the mind as an external event or as a separate person.
2. Precede BDD thoughts by the phrase "I'm having the thought that...." Patients learn the difference between thinking, "My nose is huge and makes me look awful," which sounds like a statement of fact, and "I'm having the thought that my nose is huge and makes me look awful."
3. Say the thought in different tones, use silly voices, and pretend you are a television reporter or radio announcer, or sing the thought.
4. Look around your office and notice that every single object or aspect can be evaluated in a negative way. Teach patients that *everything* can be evaluated.

Acceptance in ACT refers to the practice of allowing unpleasant internal experiences (urges, feelings, sensations) to exist without trying to push or suppress them. Struggling with them only increases your attention to them rather than allowing them to come and go. BDD patients can benefit in a number of ways by learning to experience unpleasant internal experiences and not engage in typical escape, avoidance, checking, or improving behaviors. Having the unpleasant thought "my hair must look awful" does not have to result in leaving a party or looking in the mirror. Building acceptance skills can also increase willingness to engage in exposure therapy exercises.

Values, as discussed above, are things you care most about. They guide your life, determine how you want to live, and shape what you want to be. In ACT, the goal is to help individuals engage in behavior that fits with their values. *Committed action* is the idea that acting toward your values will lead to a meaningful and fulfilling life. Exercises for values can include values clarification worksheets, which are readily available in workbooks on ACT, such as *Get out of your mind and into your life* by Steven Hayes (Hayes, 2005).

4.4.4 Addressing Trauma and Loss

Trauma, abuse, and loss, especially if the patient is exhibiting posttraumatic stress disorder (PTSD) symptoms, require additional treatment. Even if a history of childhood or adolescent bullying and teasing has not led to PTSD symptoms, these traumatic memories may need to be addressed separately. If the patient brings up early memories on multiple occasions, then the clinician should take note and explore the idea of trauma treatment to help the patient resolve and process these memories. Prolonged exposure therapy (Foa & Rothbaum, 1998) and cognitive processing therapy (Resick, Monson, & Chard, 2016) are two options for addressing trauma. Cognitive processing therapy is a type of CBT typically conducted over 12 sessions aimed at helping patients identify and restructure unhelpful beliefs related to a trauma. Cognitive processing consists of psychoeducation, writing detailed accounts of the traumatic experiences along with the identification and challenge of unhelpful thoughts and patterns of avoidance of thoughts and feelings connected to the trauma. Imagery rescripting, detailed below in the section that follows, can also be implemented for traumatic memories and images from the past.

Interestingly, many patients who have developed BDD due to a change in their appearance resulting from aging (hair loss, wrinkles), an accident (breaking their nose, car accident), or a medical condition (psoriasis, vitiligo, cystic acne) frequently describe feelings of loss and trauma. They may report loss of their youth, a loss of feeling normal, a loss of joy that comes from feeling unattractive, a loss of identity, or lost opportunities for dating and intimacy. These core and intermediate beliefs should be addressed and processed in treatment using CT techniques.

Imagery Rescripting

Imagery rescripting therapy (ImRs) is a therapeutic technique designed to address distressing images connected to early memories of traumatic events. It was initially designed for PTSD (Smucker et al., 1995), but it has also been utilized for other conditions, including BDD, with some success (Ritter & Stangier, 2015; Wilson et al., 2016).

BDD individuals struggle with a distorted self-image. Some research suggests that this negative body image may be connected to early aversive experiences given the reported history of abuse (Didie et al., 2006; Neziroglu et al., 2006) and appearance- and competency-related teasing (Buhlmann et al., 2007; Weingarden & Renshaw, 2016; Weingarden et al., 2017) that are often recalled vividly (Buhlmann et al., 2011). BDD individuals have also reported recurrent, detailed images of themselves from an observer perspective frequently connected to early memories of teasing and bullying and self-consciousness with adolescence body changes (Osman et al., 2004).

The goal of imagery rescripting is to create an alternate meaning for the image and to disconnect those early images from the patient's current image and/or current self-view. Imagery rescripting should be used in the following circumstances (Veale & Neziroglu, 2010):

1. When patients have intrusive images of themselves that are linked to early traumatic memories of abuse, teasing, bullying, self-consciousness, rejection, or humiliation.
2. For memories identified as important in the development of self-view. Patients may not have specific images, but they may have negative memories that have become linked to their body image.
3. Images that are connected to the onset of a negative picture in one's mind. This may not be an aversive event, but a memory of looking at oneself in the mirror and noticing the perceived flaw for the first time.

> Imagery rescripting is a technique for addressing traumatic memories

The following are suggested steps in applying imagery rescription in BDD (Veale & Neziroglu, 2010; Wilson et al., 2016).

Assessment
1. Identify the presence of any recurrent mental image the patient experiences when they are distressed about their appearance. The image may involve other sensory experiences including how one's body felt (tightness, heaviness). Identify images the person has when they are *not* in the mirror.
2. Ask the patient to describe the image. Is it from an observer's perspective or a self-perspective?
3. What are the assumptions and beliefs about the imagery? What does that mean about you? About your relationship with others?
4. Conduct an understanding of the connection between this mental picture with past experiences. Is there a particular incident or memory connected to this image? Collect historical data about how the person felt about themselves during that time. Were there any other relevant events occurring during that time that impacted the patient?
5. Identify if anything triggers (situations, emotions, cognitions, behaviors) the image. Does it pop up unexpectedly?
6. Assess the level of distress associated with the image.

Reliving the Experience
Step 1 is from the younger self's perspective: Ask the patient to revisit the traumatic memory from the age the patient was when they first experienced it. Clarify and confirm that the meaning of that event is one identified earlier. Identify comments made by others about appearance. Identify what the child would have needed in that moment.

Step 2 is from the adult's self-perspective: The second stage is to ask the patient to revisit the childhood memory as an adult and describe the same memory from an adult's point of view. The goal is for the adult to provide compassion and care for their younger self's needs and to assess what help the younger self needs. It is to also to provide a different perspective on the event, established using cognitive restructuring. Assess how the adult self sees the younger self; is the adult compassionate or judgmental toward the younger self? Encourage your patient to provide empathy and support to themselves.

Imagery Rescripting
Step 3 is memory rescripting: The patient revisits the memory as a child with the adult also in the room to rescue and help them. The younger self can ask the adult regarding what else they need to have done for them in that situation.

4.4.5 Addressing Skin Picking and Hair Pulling

Skin picking is a common symptom in BDD and can vary, but is generally found in approximately one third of the population (Grant et al., 2006). Clinicians should evaluate skin-picking behavior as it relates to the BDD as well as any other functions of the behavior. Typically, skin concerns are the main reason for skin picking, with the aim of improving skin, removing blemishes, and achieving smoothness. The behavior can morph into a habit or an emotion regulation strategy beyond the BDD. In this case, habit reversal (Azrin & Nunn, 1973) can be implemented in addition to the other techniques. Unfortunately, the damage from skin picking leads to further appearance distress. This in turn triggers more skin picking in attempts to inspect or "fix" the damage done by skin picking. Inspection can be visual or tactile by frequently feeling the area for bumps, scabs, and scars.

Similar to skin picking, some individuals with BDD may engage in *hair pulling* (trichotillomania), either as a comorbid condition or as appearance based to achieve smooth, hair-free body parts. Hair pulling can also morph into a habit, even if its initial aim is appearance improvement.

The following steps are recommended to address repetitive skin picking and hair pulling:

1. *Self-monitoring:* Ask the patient to record all instances of picking or pulling, over the course of the week, with time of day, how long they engaged in the behavior, a rating for their urge (1–10), and the trigger (situation, thoughts, and emotions).
2. *Assess and address motivation for change:* Explain the self-defeating cycle, and how skin picking worsens rather than improves appearance.
3. *What are the consequences of picking or pulling?* How did they feel after doing it? Did the behavior lead to more episodes? Is there a feeling of satisfaction at having removed something from the body?
4. *Remove access to any implements used to pick or pull:* This can include pins and tweezers. Supervised use of tweezers can be allowed if family members are able to help.
5. *Target the cognitions:* both those related to appearance ("I need perfectly smooth skin to be attractive") and those specific to picking ("I feel better when I do it," "I will stop after I pick at one pimple," and/or "I'll stop tomorrow").
6. *Identify and address sensory triggers:* These may include feeling the area, experiencing tightening, tingling, or itching. Strategies to reduce those triggers may include wearing gloves or using soothing lotions or ice to reduce the sensations.
7. *Make it hard to pick or pull, by introducing competing responses:* This can include wearing gloves, long sleeves or pants if picking arms/legs, or making a fist when the urge occurs.
8. *Identify and separate the sensory need to fidget versus the sensations on the skin:* Help the patient create a toolbox of things to fidget or play with, which may include silly putty, fidget toys, or hair brushes with strong bristles. Identify if certain activities are more satisfying than others, such as picking lint off a sweater or playing with the fringe of a scarf.
9. *Problem solve ways to alter environmental influences:* Items in the environment such as mirrors or lighting can be altered. Or the patient may sit in a different chair that does not have an arm to lean on or have a family member in the bathroom when engaging in necessary grooming.

10. *Identify the emotion regulation benefits of picking or pulling:* Does the patient engage in the behavior when stressed, bored, anxious, or excited? Develop skills for healthier coping with these emotions.

4.4.6 Self-Surgery

In some circumstances, patients with BDD become so disturbed by their appearance that they engage in more dramatic methods to improve their appearance. These do-it-yourself surgeries can result in significant and permanent bodily damage. Examples include breaking one's nose using a hammer, injecting oneself with a substance, or slicing out skin blemishes. Patients who become increasingly distressed and cannot afford cosmetic surgery or have been turned down by a surgeon, may resort to these solutions (Veale, 2000). Do-it-yourself surgeries also occur in the presence of significant disgust and excessive mirror checking (Veale & Neziroglu, 2010). Clinicians who believe a patient is at risk for significant self-imposed self-injury should consider hospitalization and collaborate with psychiatrists to assess risk and interventions.

4.4.7 Addressing Poor Quality of Life

Symptom reduction is not often sufficient for patients to experience a true improvement in their life quality. They may engage in fewer rituals and have fewer appearance-related obsessions, but still not experience meaning or joy in their lives. Patients often discontinue treatment after achieving symptom reduction, before they can truly address these secondary goals. It is therefore important to bring up the concept of quality of life with patients once their symptoms have begun to improve. This is a good time to review short- and long-term life goals, incorporate more meaningful and important experiences in life, and move toward richer and deeper relationships. Patients with severe BDD may not have had many intimate friendships or relationships, may have missed academic and/or occupational opportunities, and may have avoided vacations for years. Clinicians should help patients develop a plan to achieve these goals in order to develop a meaningful life. ACT and DBT both incorporate a commitment to building meaningful lives, and exercises from these modules can be revisited in sessions. Patients at this stage may benefit from action-oriented steps during the session, such as registering for college classes, building a resume, or signing up for an online dating service. Action steps toward building a better quality of life may be a crucial variable in reducing future relapses and setbacks.

> Improving quality of life aids in maintaining treatment gains

4.4.8 Maintenance and Relapse Prevention

For many patients, relapse prevention requires ongoing deliberate exposure exercises as well as reviewing their CT skills on a regular basis (see Appendix 10). Ongoing treatment on a reduced schedule for 6 months to a year after symptom improvement is recommended. Severity and functional

> Ongoing treatment to prevent relapse is recommended for up to a year after symptom improvement

impairment at onset of treatment can guide a relapse prevention plan. A step-down schedule can be helpful, with sessions first on a twice a month basis and then a monthly basis until the patient has successfully managed a variety of environmental triggers and life circumstances. If the patient decides to discontinue medication during this time, ongoing therapy should be continued. Family involvement in developing a collaborative relapse prevention plan is also important, as loved ones may be the first to notice any slight reemergence of symptoms, and they can facilitate booster sessions as needed. Relapse prevention strategies have led to better maintenance and continued improvement when compared with no further treatment (McKay, 1999; McKay et al., 1997).

4.5 Problems Carrying Out the Treatments

Engagement and adherence are frequent treatment obstacles. In the case of BDD, clinicians, more often than not, need to weave in alternate treatment methods and anticipate a longer time frame to achieve progress. Techniques such as goal clarification, MI, and family engagement are not optional strategies, as they might be in other disorders. Those techniques should not be rushed in the initial stages of treatment. Often, even patients with better insight will waver in treatment adherence or may struggle with suicidal ideation.

The following is a list of the most common obstacles to the treatment of BDD: (1) high overvalued ideation leading to lack of desire to engage in treatment, (2) suicidal risk, (3) pursuing cosmetic surgery simultaneously with psychological treatment, (4) nonadherence to treatment, (5) family accommodation, and (6) therapist variables.

Interventions for many of these complications have already been covered in the previous sections of this chapter, as they are more often the norm than the exception in this population. High overvalued ideation can be addressed via CT, incorporation of values-based strategies, focusing on patients' suffering and distress about appearance, and therapists' flexibility in treatment delivery.

Suicidality and the desire for cosmetic surgery are addressed below, as both place inordinate pressure on the clinician to manage these critical factors with a patient who is not engaging in treatment in order to address the very problem leading to these high-risk behaviors.

4.5.1 Addressing Desire for Cosmetic Surgery

The desire and active pursuit of cosmetic surgery often places a time-sensitive burden on the clinician to intervene and stop the behavior. Family members are often unable to halt the process or are caught up in unhealthy ways. Patients may enter treatment with a prior decision to pursue cosmetic surgery. At times, family members will have agreed to pay for surgery in exchange for a trial of therapy, assuming therapy will obviate the need for the surgery. The patient's motivation, in these cases, may be to tolerate therapy long enough to satisfy their family's expectations, without a genuine intention to engage in treatment. Patients may even pressure the therapist to support their decision and convince family members to agree to support cosmetic surgery. This places clinicians in a very difficult bind. We recommend a firm yet flexible approach, expressing a genuine desire to understand the patient's desire for cosmetic surgery, yet maintaining an unwavering message against cosmetic surgery. Clinicians should encourage and welcome discussions, as these conversations will not reinforce surgery, but can provide an opportunity to keep the patient engaged in treatment. If the patient seeks cosmetic consultations during the course of therapy, the clinician should consider accompanying them to these appointments, as they often misinterpret the surgeon's opinion and advice.

It is not easy to engage patients in discussions regarding their need for cosmetic surgery and at the same time present data that argue against it. The following are some specific suggestions on approaching these conversations to help the patient make a wise decision about surgery:

1. Educate the patient about the psychiatric and psychological literature providing evidence for why surgery is contraindicated for BDD. Even if the patient disputes the validity of the data or applicability to their particular situation, it is important to present a credible and scientific rationale. Patients may disagree but still reflect on the information.
2. Discuss the possibility of a discrepancy between the surgeon's understanding versus the patient's understanding of what exactly needs to be altered physically. Discuss how difficult it is for a surgeon to share their mental representation of an ideal self. Ask the patient the following questions: Did the surgeon demonstrate an understanding of your needs? Has the surgeon expressed the ability and probability of producing the desired results? Does the surgeon explain the physical characteristics in the same way you do? Does the surgeon agree with your perception of the flaw? Or are they agreeing to perform the surgery regardless of the need to improve that body part?
3. Similar to the above recommendation, discuss the likelihood of achieving the perfect outcome or getting exactly the change your patient wants from surgery. Is the expectation for surgery achievable? Does the medical field have the tools and ability to create your desired outcome? For patients who have had some prior surgery, this might be more believable, since they have continued to feel dissatisfied and in fact may be worse off than they were presurgery.
4. A fourth angle is to examine the psychological risk if they do not achieve the desired outcome. Ask them how they imagine coping with a less-than-ideal outcome? Discuss the level of treatment progress and the risk of a depressive episode, increase in symptoms, and risk of suicide that can occur. Psychological postsurgery complications are just as critical as any medical complications.
5. Point out the level of medical risk one is taking, especially for procedures that are particularly risky or are performed by only a handful of medical experts – for example, limb lengthening to be taller, or jaw masseter muscle reduction. Is the patient clear on the recovery period and the amount of discomfort and pain? How will they cope with their postsurgery appearance, which may include very visible scars, skin dis-

coloration, and swelling. How will they cope with anticipatory anxiety and uncertainty for the weeks or possibly months until they can judge the surgery outcome?

Ultimately, patients may choose to proceed with cosmetic surgery despite your best effort to dissuade them. In these cases, it is important to make every effort to collaborate with family members and any other mental health professionals involved in the patient's care, as well as the cosmetic surgeon to prepare for possible postsurgery emotional reactions. If a patient is not on psychotropic medication previous to the surgery, strongly advise them to seek a consultation with a psychiatrist or psychopharmacologist with expertise in BDD. There have been instances in which patients have sued their surgeon or become violent or hostile. These are possible crises that clinicians need to be prepared for and seek supervision to manage well.

4.5.2 Addressing Suicidality

> Structured suicide measures and protocols can be incorporated to manage risk

Suicidality becomes an unfortunate and intimidating clinical variable in treating BDD patients. Assessment of ideation, urges, and plan is recommended every session. Formalized assessment instruments may also be included to track suicidal ideation and intent, such as the Sheehan Suicidality Tracking Scale (S-STS; Sheehan et al., 2014).

Three structured protocols for suicidal ideation have shown the most positive treatment outcomes (Jobes et al., 2015). *Cognitive therapy for suicidal patients* (CT-SP) is a manualized approach based on Aaron Beck's CBT model (Brown et al., 2005). DBT (Linehan, 1993) has also shown benefit in addressing suicidal ideation, although most of the research outcome is based on female research participants (Jobes et al., 2015). *Collaborative assessment and management of suicidality* (CAMS; Jobes, 2012) is another validated treatment option that emphasizes a philosophy of collaboration, nonjudgment, and empathy. Clinicians may want to consider suspending CBT for BDD and follow a structured suicide protocol when suicidal ideation and risk is increasing despite treating the BDD. Hospitalization and psychopharmacological interventions should be considered to manage suicide risk.

4.5.3 Nonadherence to Treatment

Several strategies for initial treatment engagement have been highlighted in the beginning of this chapter, including goal clarification and MI. Nonadherence can occur at any stage of the process, and these strategies should be revisited when they occur. For example, the patient may tolerate CT, but then avoid and resist ERP. They may not reveal active pursuit of cosmetic surgery consultations or resist the reduction in BDD safety seeking and repetitive behaviors.

Clinicians should approach these obstacles from a position of genuine interest in a nonjudgmental manner in identifying reasons for noncompliance. Meeting the patient where they are in their change process will can help reduce chances of patient termination, and limit arguing with the patient or lecturing about the benefits of applying the recommended strategies. Clinicians, instead, should approach nonadherence by conducting a proper functional analysis to elucidate the cause of the resistance. For example, family accommodation may be reinforcing reassurance seeking, necessitating family sessions to identify dynamics and support families to make the necessary changes. Shame and fear of clinician judgment may be a factor in not revealing certain rituals. Homework compliance can be addressed with home visits to encourage generalization of treatment gains outside session. The clinician may need to problem solve to overcome obstacles for the patient, such as their not finding opportunities to practice, their need to balance other responsibilities, or confusion regarding the purpose of the assigned homework.

4.5.4 Family Involvement and Accommodation

Obsessive-compulsive and related disorders, including BDD, OCD, and hoarding disorder, often directly impact family members. Individuals with these disorders often seek direct involvement in rituals, seek reassurance, or require assistance to complete daily tasks due to impairment levels. Often family involvement can exacerbate and enable the symptoms of the sufferer. The OCD literature therefore has extensive research into the reaction and family response styles and their impact on treatment outcome. In OCD, there are two typical response styles: *accommodation* and *antagonism* (Van Noppen et al., 1997), which family members may vacillate between. Accommodation refers to family members supporting and facilitating their loved one's rituals and avoidance, while an antagonistic style refers to reacting with criticism, blame, and hostility.

In BDD, the family is typically very involved due to the distress and functional impairment that often accompanies the disorder. Family members are often in turmoil and confused about the diagnosis, especially with expressed depression and suicidal ideation. Family members are also likely to be the ones to initiate treatment for their loved one. Their ongoing involvement is almost always recommended in order to enhance treatment adherence and outcome. Family members can benefit from psychoeducation, structured guidance on how to respond to rituals, and ongoing support. Clinicians can suggest regular family meetings in addition to individual therapy, to address the needs of the patient and the family. At times, a referral for family therapy may also be beneficial. In these cases, the family therapist should have a solid understanding of BDD.

4.6 Multicultural Issues in Treatment

International prevalence studies in various countries, including Germany, Brazil, and Turkey, suggest that BDD is found globally. Core clinical characteristics, age of onset, course, sex ratio, and symptomatology remain fairly consistent across cultures, further supporting the neurobiological basis of BDD. Despite these similarities, little is known about the differences in BDD expression.

BDD is found worldwide

Sociocultural ideals, including standards of beauty, gender roles, and racial influences all impact body image ideals and concerns. There is some evidence that culture-specific factors could create variability in body parts of concern and related behaviors. For example, in some Asian cultures, light skin is a highly valued trait historically connected to the lifestyle of the wealthy. In Japan, eyelid concerns are more common than in Western cultures. In African American women, hair and skin tone concerns are influenced by European ideals of beauty (Awad et al., 2015). Studies have shown that African American women generally positively endorse a curvy and larger body type than White and Latina women (Gordon et al., 2010). These are just some examples of the variability and cultural influences on standards of beauty. There is a paucity of treatment outcome research investigating how cultural influences influence treatment outcome.

According to the 2018 statistics from the International Society of Aesthetic Plastic Surgery (ISAPS), the US had the most nonsurgical procedures (botulinum toxin, hyaluronic acid, hair removal) in the world, while Brazil leads the world in surgical procedures (breast augmentation, liposuction, and eyelid surgery). When the total number of surgical and nonsurgical procedures are considered, the top five ranked countries in order are the US, Brazil, Mexico, Germany, and India. This is presumably influenced by accessibility, cost, societal standards of beauty, and levels of body dissatisfaction.

Clinicians treating BDD should identify and discuss culture-specific influences on body image beliefs and how they influence BDD symptoms. Cultural sensitivity also extends to patients' comfort in sharing personal clinical information, expectations and beliefs about psychological treatment, willingness to involve family members, and shame about having a mental illness.

4.7 Summary

Treatment for BDD often requires an intensive approach incorporating adjunct treatment modules to supplement standard CBT. Clinicians should pay close attention to trauma, suicidality, and elevated overvalued ideation, as these can often impact treatment outcomes.

5

Case Vignettes

This chapter will provide case examples to illustrate the variety of clinical presentations in body dysmorphic disorder (BDD). Vignettes will include detailed assessments modeling the recommended steps given in Chapter 4, followed by a synopsis of treatment.

5.1 Case Vignette 1: Post Accident Preoccupation With Nose

Janice, aged 49, was a married high school teacher with a 17-year-old son. She sought treatment for BDD after an unfortunate accident in her home. Her clinical history consisted of a mild preoccupation with skin after developing acne in her teenage years. She sought dermatological treatment at age 17 and recalled anxiety and some social avoidance during college. After 6 months of weekly therapy and a trial of medication, Janice went on to attend graduate school and successfully worked full time. During her pregnancy, she developed acne again which led to excessive preoccupation, mild depression, and mirror checking. She responded well to therapy and a second trial of medication after giving birth to her child. Her clinical history was uneventful after the birth of her son. She cited mild concerns about her overall appearance that did not interfere with functioning.

Approximately 9 months ago, Janice accidentally bruised her nose on a kitchen cabinet door resulting in swelling and discomfort for many weeks. She subsequently became convinced that her nose had healed in an irregular manner, looking larger and crooked. Her concern escalated to a daily preoccupation resulting in multiple hours in front of a mirror, depression, difficulty getting out of bed on weekends, and avoidance of social activities. She expressed anger and self-blame for injuring her nose. Janice sought multiple appointments with her physician who told her that she had fully healed. She had been researching cosmetic surgeons for a second opinion, believing an expert could easily observe the damage. Janice recently began a trial of antidepressant medication after struggling for months.

Janice was ambivalent toward a BDD diagnosis since she believed that her problem was based on real damage and not an "imagined" flaw. She had read about the diagnosis and did not believe it applied to her circumstances. She reported recent depression and hopelessness. Janice believed that the accident had taken away her youth and beauty. Janice had a supportive husband and family, and she denied any significant environmental stressors. She did express sadness at her son's upcoming transition from high school to college as he was beginning his senior year of high school. Janice agreed to engage in treatment in order to address what she defined as trauma from the accident.

Baseline Assessment

Structured Measures
1. Yale-Brown Obsessive-Compulsive Scale for BDD (BDD-YBOCS): Total score of 30, which is in the severe range.
2. Beck Depression Inventory – Second Edition (BDI-II): Total score of 27, which is in the moderate range.
3. Overvalued Ideas Scale: Belief that "my nose is misshapen and I am unattractive, look old, and deformed." Her total score was a 6 indicating a moderate degree of belief.

Suicidality
Janice reported passive suicidal ideation without intent or a plan. She expressed clear reasons she would not act on ideation, including religious beliefs and love for her family. She denied any previous history of suicidal thoughts.

Clinical Assessment

Description of body part: Janice described her nose as deformed. Specifically, she felt it had widened, had changed color to be slightly redder, and had become slightly angled toward her right.

Thoughts and beliefs: When looking in the mirror, Janice saw herself as deformed, with a crooked misshapen nose, which made her look old and ugly. She felt that she had lost herself and could not recognize herself in the mirror. She longed to have her old face back and believed that her life would never be the same again unless her nose could go back to its previous appearance. She believed that her family and friends were not being truthful when they repeatedly told her that she looked the same as she always had. She was not as concerned about other people's judgments as much as her own loss of attractiveness. On the bell curve, Janice rated her overall appearance as very low average due to her injury, when she previously felt she was above average. She rated her nose as very unattractive and deformed.

Janice's Intermediate BDD Beliefs
1. Looking young is the only way to be attractive.
2. I can't be happy unless I look the way I used to.

Janice's Core Beliefs
1. There's something wrong with me.
2. I'm not good enough.

Janice noticed that although her mood had not shifted greatly, she was able to intellectually grasp and acknowledge the value of challenging automatic negative thoughts. She continued to complete thought records and engage in cognitive therapy in addition to planning for exposure therapy. In Session 7, Janice expressed a desire to attempt some exposure exercises. Sessions 8 onwards consisted of exposure exercises with debriefing to discuss shifts in her cognitions. Intermediate and core beliefs were addressed in these later sessions. Values clarification exercises helped Janice address her emphasis on youth and beauty.

The therapist incorporated conversations to help Janice address her fear of aging, which was being exacerbated by her son's approaching 18th birthday and college plans. Janice was also taught mirror retraining and asked to practice for homework. She was asked to record herself during homework mirror retraining in order to ensure she did not engage in critical, judgmental descriptions.

Janice continued intensive treatment for 4 weeks at which time her BDD-YBOCS score was reduced from a rating of 30 to 20, and her BDI-II was reduced from a rating of 27 to 18. Her Overvalued Ideas Scale score was reduced from 6 to 4. She was instructed to refrain from any checking after she was dressed in the morning. She had also refrained from researching surgeons and had reduced taking photographs of herself to one a day in the morning.

Sessions were slowly reduced to twice a week for 60 minutes for the next month and then to once weekly. During this period, Janice was able to engage in many of her target exercises on her hierarchy but was unable to post photos of herself without makeup. It was recommended that Janice continue weekly sessions for continued reinforcement of gains for an additional 3 months and then reduce those to twice-monthly for maintenance and relapse prevention. During this later period, Janice was able to go on vacation with her family successfully and experienced less anxiety while attending a wedding.

Treatment Schedule
1. Four weeks of treatment at three times a week for 2 hrs.
2. Four weeks of treatment at two times a week for 60 minutes.
3. Three months of weekly sessions.
4. Ongoing sessions twice a month to slowly reduce to monthly.

Compulsive and Avoidance Behaviors
1. *Compulsive behaviors:*
   a. Mirror checking; in the past, mirror avoidance
   b. Pressing on her nose with her fingers in an attempt to reshape it
   c. Seeking reassurance from her husband
   d. Wearing makeup to try to reduce shadows on her face to make her nose appear thinner
   e. Checking her reflection in windows in her classroom
   f. Researching cosmetic surgery
   g. Comparing herself with other people who had had accidents and damage to their nose
   h. Comparing her nose with that of other people throughout the day.
2. *Avoidance:*
   Janice was able to go to work, but avoided being in the staff room at lunch. She also stopped much of her socializing. She felt very uncomfortable in crowded, brightly lit places, and did not let anyone sit to her

right, believing the crooked shape was more evident from that angle. Otherwise, she was able to go to work and felt comfortable with her students.

Functional Analysis of Mirror Checking
1. In the morning before work or anytime she had to leave home. Prolonged period of checking in the morning for approximately 30 minutes. Checking involved posing in different angles to check for swelling and size.
2. Stayed before the mirror until she achieved a "good image" of herself.
3. She checked at night before bed to look for any changes from morning to night.
4. Use of extra lighting in bathroom.
5. Pressing bridge of her nose to make it thinner in the mirror. It had become habitual for her to touch her nose throughout the day.
6. Mirror checking also triggered by seeing women with a certain facial structure or when comparing with others.
7. Mirror checking triggered from a sensory experience of tingling in her nose.
8. At times felt nose looked better, and at other times worse. Continued to look to see herself better.

Janice's Exposure Hierarchy
90 Posting a photo of herself on social media without makeup (at the beach, park)
80 Taking photographs and posting photographs on social media
75 Going to work with less makeup
70 Seeing friends and family who have not seen her since the accident
60 Having lunch with colleagues at work in the teachers' lounge
55 Going to a store without makeup on
50 Shopping for makeup with salesperson's advice and help
45 Sitting in clinic waiting room with people to her right
40 Therapist sitting next to Janice on her right side in a brighter room
30 Therapist sitting next to Janice on her right side in a dark room
20 Walking around in a public store

Etiological Variables

Janice described her childhood as normal and happy. She did recall that her mother would frequently comment on other's clear complexion and beautiful skin tone. Her family psychiatric history consisted of a paternal uncle with obsessive-compulsive disorder, and her father had episodes of mild depression throughout his life. Janice described herself as a perfectionistic in her work life.

Treatment

Janice agreed to intensive treatment based on her level of distress and daily functioning. Therapy was scheduled for 90 minutes three times a week. Janice had been able to continue working full time but agreed to increase treatment frequency if she experienced worsening symptoms or work impairment. Sessions 1 through 2 consisted of rapport building, psychoeducation, assessment, and going through a typical weekday and a typical weekend. The therapist also began building a basic hierarchy of feared and avoided situations. Janice was motivated for treatment despite her ambivalence about the BDD diagnosis. She displayed sufficient insight that her behavior was not helpful, even though she believed it was a justifiable response to her circumstances. Janice was given homework worksheets to track her daily mirror checking in the first session. Her husband came in for brief periods in each of these sessions to learn about the diagnosis and provide his perspective on his wife's daily symptoms. They were coached on the negative impact of reassurance seeking and general conversations about appearance. In Session 2, the therapist engaged Janice in holistic perceptual retraining exercises for neutral images.

In Session 3 she was taught cognitive therapy and was given thought records to complete for homework. She also completed worksheets on goal setting and values clarification. Janice was instructed to begin response prevention exercises by systematically reducing her mirror checking to 10 minutes in the morning as well as reducing the number of times she pressed and touched her nose throughout the day. Sessions 4–6 continued cognitive therapy in-session by reviewing thought records, identifying cognitive distortions, and introducing the concept of intermediate and core beliefs. Janice was able to reduce her morning mirror check to 15 minutes, but continued to check her reflection on other surfaces and research possible surgical solutions for her nose.

5.2 Case Vignette 2: Preoccupation With Facial Shape and Muscle Dysmorphia

Daniel was a 22-year-old single man living with his parents and younger sister. Daniel became self-conscious about his appearance at age 15, when he lagged behind his friends in growth and puberty. He was teased by his classmates and given nicknames regarding his small stature throughout high school. His family reported that Daniel became irritable and withdrawn, intermittently struggling with school attendance despite being bright and academically high achieving. During high school, Daniel began to lift weights excessively and do stretching exercises with the belief that it would help him grow taller and more muscular.

Daniel graduated high school and enrolled in an out-of-state university, completing 2 years successfully. In his third year of classes, he experienced an exacerbation of symptoms necessitating a medical withdrawal from college. His parents first learned about his BDD upon his return home. Daniel also revealed that his recent breakup with a girl had led to increasing suicidal ideation and symptom worsening. Daniel's parents immediately sought a psychiatric and psychological evaluation.

Daniel was preoccupied with the shape of his chin, his overall muscularity, and most recently a fear of thinning hair. He had recently started researching cosmetic surgery and had scheduled a consultation without his parents' knowledge. During the initial psychological evaluation, he expressed significant reluctance to engage in treatment and did not accept the diagnosis of BDD, but came to the consultation due to pressure from his parents. Daniel endorsed significant depression symptoms since his recent relationship breakup. His ex-girlfriend had begun dating an attractive athlete soon after the breakup, reinforcing his belief that his appearance was connected to the failed relationship. Daniel stopped attending his classes and slept much of the day. Upon return to his home, he continued to experience a sleep reversal schedule. His only activity consisted of daily exercise at the gym.

Baseline Assessment

Structured Measures
1. Yale-Brown Obsessive Compulsive Scale for BDD (BDD-YBOCS): Total score of 34, which is in the severe range.
2. Beck Depression Inventory – Second Edition (BDI-II): Total score of 45, which is in the severe range.
3. Overvalued Ideas Scale: Belief that "I will always be alone because my chin is recessed and does not look masculine." His total score of 8 indicated a high degree of belief in his BDD thought.

Suicidality
Although Daniel had episodes of suicidal ideation since age 17, he had no history of suicidal attempts. He indicated that his ideation might increase if he was prevented from cosmetic surgery. He expressed a strong belief that improving his appearance was the only way to be successful in life. He denied

a specific suicide plan, but had thought of possible ways to kill himself in the past, including jumping off a bridge or a drug overdose.

Clinical Assessment

Description of body part: Daniel expressed dissatisfaction with three aspects of his appearance. His primary focus was on the shape of his chin, which he described as feminine looking. Daniel desired a strong and masculine jawline. He also believed his chest and abdomen were not muscular enough. Recently, he worried about thinning hair after noticing that his forehead seemed larger and more exposed. His previous concern about height had improved after he had entered college and reached an above-average height.

Thoughts and Beliefs: Daniel described himself as generally unattractive and feminine looking. He predicted that women would always reject him unless he had cosmetic surgery. He could not accept looking the way he did, and he believed that it would be intolerable and unacceptable to him. Daniel rated his overall appearance as very low average due to his facial structure and body shape. He rated his face as 3 out of 10 and his body as 4 out of 10. Daniel reported that he would not be satisfied unless he was an 8 out of 10.

Daniel's Intermediate BDD Beliefs
1. People should improve their appearance if they can.
2. Attractive people are happier and more successful.
3. Masculine appearance is critical for social success and approval.

Daniel's Core Beliefs
1. I'm inadequate.
2. I'm unlovable.
3. People can't be trusted.

Compulsive and Avoidance Behaviors
1. *Compulsive behaviors:*
   a. Comparing himself to others in person and social media
   b. Mirror checking
   c. Researching cosmetic surgery
   d. Daily exercise at a gym for 2 hrs with a strict routine
   e. Wearing a hat to hide his hair
   f. Avoiding brightly lit and crowded places
   g. Holding his hand on his chin in public
   h. Measuring the size of his chin
   i. Measuring his chest and biceps for gain in mass
   j. Rigidity in daily diet
   k. Taking 100s of selfies to get the perfect one, but not being able to achieve it
2. *Avoidance:*
   a. Avoidance of socializing, including bars and restaurants
   b. Avoidance of academic classes and peer interactions
   c. Avoidance of having photographs taken and posting on social media

Functional Analysis of Mirror Checking

Daniel had had episodes of both mirror avoidance and mirror checking since the age of 15. At the time of treatment, he was engaging in regular mirror checking.

1. He checked in the morning and throughout the day. He used his bathroom mirror along with a handheld mirror to check his profile.
2. He used a full-length mirror to check for an increase in muscle mass in his torso.
3. He had become increasingly depressed after mirror checking as he believed his exercise routine had not resulted in satisfactory muscle gain.
4. Mirror checking was also triggered by seeing attractive people and photos on social media

Daniel's Exposure Hierarchy for Chin Concerns

90 Posting photos of himself on social media with profile visible
80 Going to a bar with friends and sitting side by side with profile noticeable
70 Sitting next to an attractive woman with profile noticeable
60 Engaging in conversation with attractive women without hand on chin
50 Interacting with friends without hand on chin
40 Sitting next to stranger with profile noticeable
30 Interacting with strangers without hand on chin

Daniel's Exposure Hierarchy for Muscularity

100 Taking his shirt off at the beach
90 Posting photos of himself at beach or swimming pool without a shirt on
80 Posting photos of himself on social media with form-fitting T-shirt
70 Skipping a day at the gym
60 Skipping one exercise at the gym
50 Using less weight or fewer exercises at the gym
40 Wearing a form-fitting T-shirt around friends
30 Wearing a form-fitting T-shirt around a stranger
20 Wearing a form-fitting shirt in session and office

Etiological Variables

Daniel had a history of being teased in the ninth grade that continued until he graduated high school. He reported vivid memories of being teased in front of a girl he liked, as well as in the locker room during physical education classes. He reported that although most of the teasing was meant to be humorous by his friends, he experienced feelings of embarrassment and humiliation. Daniel had a family history of clinical depression and OCD on both his maternal and paternal side.

Treatment

Daniel reluctantly entered treatment after his parents agreed to consider paying for a cosmetic surgery consultation in exchange for his participation in therapy. He agreed to four weeks of intensive sessions, five times a week for 3 hrs, as long as his sessions did not interfere with his exercise schedule. Family therapy was also recommended to address the surgery conflict. Daniel did not initially agree to a psychiatric consultation as recommended.

Initial treatment goals were to (1) increase treatment engagement, (2) decrease suicidal ideation and depression, (3) encourage a psychiatric consultation, (5) decrease familial conflict, and (6) parental psychoeducation and coaching.

Individual therapy began with psychoeducation about BDD and motivational interviewing. Although his main objective was receiving financial support for cosmetic surgery, Daniel and the therapist were able to identify his other life goals, including completing college and moving to California. He also agreed to address his recent lethargy, motivated by his desire to increase his exercise performance and efficiency. He strongly believed that surgery and other appearance-enhancing behaviors were his only option for happiness.

Suicidal ideation was assessed daily, and the Sheehan Suicidality Tracking Scale was administered weekly. Daniel continued to experience passive ideation without an escalation in desire or plans to harm himself. Suicide assessment was conducted at each session, and a safety plan was developed to address any increase in risk.

While reviewing the CBT model of BDD, Daniel disclosed his history of being teased, and he described himself as quite self-conscious in high school. He expressed continued anger about these past traumatic incidents, which had led to a mistrust of others. His recent breakup with his girlfriend contributed to his depression and hopelessness. He generally discounted the importance of these events on his self-image. He attributed his current suffering to what he clearly saw in the mirror. He believed that the mirror could not lie and that his perceptions were accurate. Global perceptual retraining was initiated to illustrate the negative impact of mirror checking and detailed processing on his perception. Daniel complied with the exercises, but held onto his initial beliefs. He was given literature to read for homework to further support the perceptual theory of BDD. The therapist continued to educate Daniel on how his beliefs, emotions, and mirror checking impacted his perceptual experiences and self-image.

The therapist first targeted Daniel's hopelessness about the future and depression in order to decrease suicidal ideation. Behavioral activation exercises were introduced, and Daniel engaged in walks at a shopping mall and park during sessions. The therapist gradually introduced cognitive therapy (CT) to challenge cognitive distortions articulated by him during these outings. The therapist only targeted beliefs that could be disputed with observed evidence and were not strongly held including that (1) everyone will notice my flaws, (2) attractive people are happier, and (3) unattractive people are alone in life. In-session CT targeted his hopelessness about the future and his relationship breakup. He believed his ex-girlfriend had rejected him based on his appearance, because she began dating someone very attractive after their breakup.

Daniel demonstrated mild cognitive shifts with these beliefs, but continued to strongly believe that his happiness and future were conditional on being satisfied with his appearance. At this point, strategies for acceptance and commitment were incorporated that targeted his concerns and values about appearance, and Daniel's depression improved somewhat, and he agreed to see one or two friends from high school. However, Daniel was unwilling to share his struggles with his friends.

Mirror checking was targeted, and Daniel was given homework to limit his morning checking to 5 minutes and to avoid certain equipment at the gym that was located near a mirror.

In the middle of the second week of treatment, unbeknownst to his therapists and parents, Daniel had a cosmetic surgery consultation for chin enhancement. The surgeon was familiar with BDD and made recommendations for therapy and a psychiatric consultation prior to surgery. Daniel became increasingly angry and refused to attend his session the following day. He disclosed his surgery consultation to his parents, and a family session was scheduled to address the issue. During the appointment, his parents and therapist were able to convince him to seek a psychiatric evaluation and continue therapy. Daniel agreed, believing it was his only way to get approved for surgery. The therapist aligned with him and discussed the benefit of an selective serotonin reuptake inhibitor (SSRI) in helping him cope with the anxiety of surgery and postsurgery recovery. Daniel consulted with a psychiatrist with an expertise in BDD and began a trial of an SSRI.

Daniel continued therapy and agreed to exposure exercises for his muscularity beliefs. He did not see the value in addressing his chin concerns, as he believed surgery was the only solution. The therapist accompanied him to the gym to observe his exercise routine and discussed gradually developing some flexibility and rotation to his exercises. Daniel agreed, as he had become increasingly exhausted by his existing rigorous exercises. He also engaged in some exposures to wear different "unflattering" clothing that he believed made him look skinny. He maintained a strict diet and made very small changes to his food intake. Mirror retraining exercises were also incorporated; first in a darkened office, and later in a brighter room. He was instructed to practice daily retraining at home.

Daniel continued treatment beyond the initially agreed upon 4 weeks if the therapist agreed to a reduced schedule. Treatment was reduced from five times a week to three times a week for 90 minutes. Daniel's SSRI dose was gradually increased, and he experienced less depression and began sleeping better. With family therapy, his parents were able to gently alter their reaction to his reassurance seeking and insistence on financial support for surgery.

Daniel was able to tolerate exposure exercises and improved his daily functioning at the end of 3 months of intensive therapy. He signed up for a course at a local community college and socialized more easily. His preoccupation with his chin and his core beliefs about appearance, however, required ongoing therapy. Daniel experienced setbacks at times leading to excessive mirror checking. Those episodes decreased in intensity and frequency with increased doses of medication and ongoing treatment. After approximately 10 months of homework and regular treatment, Daniel returned to his out-of-state university and found a therapist nearby to support him through the transition and maintain his gains.

5.3 Case Vignette 3: Preoccupation With Skin Accompanied by Skin Picking

Sophia was a 34-year-old engaged woman who sought treatment for skin picking. She was scheduled to get married in 6 months and was terrified that she would not be able to follow through with the wedding. She had been seeing a therapist for 2 years who recommended a consultation for more intensive and specialized treatment to address her symptom exacerbation.

Sophia's skin preoccupation began in middle school with the development of facial and arm acne. At age 16, she developed a mild case of cystic acne, which triggered skin picking, camouflaging, and social withdrawal. Her excessive makeup and face cleansing routine interfered with school punctuality. Because of Sophia's insistence and evident distress, her parents agreed to seek a dermatological evaluation. Sophia struggled with her body image until her acne responded to antibiotics and a prescription of isotretinoin.

Although her skin improved, Sophie had bouts of skin picking throughout college. During this time, she became excessively preoccupied with the shape of her stomach and breast size. After graduation, Sophia reported spending excessive time getting ready for her job as a paralegal at a law firm, often changing her outfit numerous times. She also engaged in a lengthy makeup routine, and she would not allow her friends or fiancé to see her without makeup. Despite these concerns, Sophia was able to work full time and maintain a social life.

Her engagement led to an increased focus on her appearance. At this time, she noticed some minor acne. Her compulsive skin picking, mirror checking, and general distress were heightened as her wedding approached. Her picking had led to some scars, which further increased her distress. Sophia willingly agreed to start treatment, demonstrating motivation and desire to improve. Her fiancé and family were supportive. Sophia had started SSRI medication 2 months prior to the psychological evaluation.

Baseline Assessment

Structured Measures
1. Yale-Brown Obsessive Compulsive Scale for BDD (BDD-YBOCS): Total score of 29, which is in the severe range.
2. Beck Depression Inventory – second edition (BDI-II): Total score of 20, which is in the moderate range.
3. Overvalued Ideas Scale: Belief that "I need perfect skin to be attractive." Her total score of 6 indicated a moderate degree of belief in her BDD thoughts.

Suicidality
Sophia denied suicidal ideation or intent. She did think life was too hard, and she wished she could escape the emotional pain she felt due to her appearance dissatisfaction.

Clinical Assessment

Description of body part: Sophia sought smooth skin, both visually and when feeling it. She hated bumps, redness, or any blemishes on her skin. She also wanted her arms to be smooth. She believed her breasts were not large enough and wished her stomach was flatter.

Thoughts and beliefs: Sophia believed that skin was a critical aspect of attractiveness. She believed people were disgusted by blemished skin. She believed that perfect skin was attainable and necessary to her happiness. She also believed if she picked her blemishes, they improved. She struggled with the belief that leaving them alone would lead to faster improvement.

Sophia's Intermediate Beliefs
1. People with good skin are more accepted.
2. I can't be happy unless I have perfect skin and a good body.

Sophia's Core Beliefs
1. I'm not good enough.

Compulsive and Avoidance Behaviors
1. *Compulsive behaviors:*
    a. Touching her face and upper arms throughout the day looking for bumps
    b. Skin picking
    c. Comparing herself with others in person and social media
    d. Mirror checking
    e. Researching dermatological creams and procedures
    f. Makeup routine requiring an hour every morning
    g. Avoiding brightly lit and crowded places
    h. Clothing choices which hid her stomach and enhanced her breasts
2. *Avoidance:*
    a. Avoidance of going out in public without makeup
    b. Avoidance of friends and fiancé seeing her without makeup
    c. Avoidance of having photographs taken or posting photos of herself on social media
    d. Avoidance of activities that would make her hot or sweat
    e. Avoidance of rooms without excessive air conditioning
    f. Avoidance of wearing red-colored clothes

Functional Analysis of Skin Picking
Antecedent Checking Behaviors and Triggers
1. Tactile checking consisted of rubbing her arms and face repeatedly seeking bumps and blemishes.
    a. Deliberately, with awareness, to check for new blemishes and to check healing of old blemishes and acne she had picked.
    b. Habitual during idle activities and intermittently throughout the day including watching television and reading.
2. Visual inspection consisted of using small makeup mirror and bathroom mirror for extended periods of time.

a. Inspecting was deliberate to check for new bumps and redness, and to also inspect healing of previously picked areas.
   b. At times, inspections occurred as a distraction from a stressful day.
3. Negative thoughts about her appearance and mental images of her ideal self triggered checking and picking.
4. Irrational beliefs regarding the positive benefits of picking. Sophia believed that picking could improve her skin by removing the infection.
5. Seeing photographs and comparing herself with others led to checking and picking.
6. Self-soothing when anxious, stressed, or bored.

Skin Picking Behavior
1. Immediately preceded by visual and tactile checking. She primarily picked bumps that were large and red that she believed were infected.
2. At times, Sophia would go directly to mirror seeking to examine areas on her face to pick, to distract and relax from a stressful day. She also picked when bored.
3. Picking episodes of face primarily occurred in the morning while applying makeup and at night before bed.
4. Tactile checking would lead to picking small bumps on arms, but these were more manageable.
5. Picking would lead to inflammation and scars and a subsequent increase.

Consequences of Picking
1. Picking created sense of accomplishment and satisfaction from removing the "infected stuff under the skin."
2. Immediate relief following picking.
3. Shame, guilt, and regret occurred soon after the picking episodes.
4. Greater distress from facial picking than arms.
5. Social avoidance increased after picking episodes.
6. Increase in mirror checking after picking episodes.

Functional Analysis of Mirror Checking
Mirror checking was primarily triggered by checking for bumps, while picking, and inspecting the results of picking. Morning mirror checking occurred for the purpose of makeup application and clothing choices. After picking episodes, she would use a small makeup mirror to check for healing and redness throughout the day.

Sophia's Exposure Hierarchy for Skin Concerns
100 No makeup at a social event (party or dinner at a restaurant)
 90 Professional photographs
 80 Exercising outdoors and getting sweaty
 70 Posting photographs on social media with no makeup
 65 Posting photos on social media with less makeup
 60 No makeup with strangers
 50 Less makeup with strangers
 40 Wearing bright-colored shirts
 30 No makeup in-session
 20 Less makeup in-session

Etiological Variables

Sophia reported that her childhood and family life were happy. In high school, she recalled one experience of being inappropriately fondled once by a neighbor. She engaged in competitive dance from a very young age until age 18.

Treatment

Sophia began treatment four times a week for 2-hr sessions. She continued to maintain full-time employmentas a paralegal. Treatment began with psychoeducation and holistic processing training. Cognitive therapy was introduced in Session 3, and she was assigned thought records to complete each session. Skin picking had become a significant cause of concern for Sophia and needed to be addressed early on in treatment. In Session 3, she was also assigned a self-monitoring skin-picking form.

In Session 4, the therapist spent half the time continuing CT and the other half introducing the comprehensive behavioral model for skin picking that included habit reversal as well comprehensive behavioral treatment for skin picking (ComB; Mansueto et al., 1999). Sophia was taught to self-monitor picking episodes to help with the assessment and awareness. Her self-monitoring forms indicated that checking and skin picking had multiple triggers and functions, as indicated in the above functional analyses. Sophia learned that her skin picking occurred in response to stress and boredom, and she became increasingly aware of her habit of rubbing and touching her face and arms during the day. The therapist incorporated her skin-picking beliefs into CT ("I need to pick to improve skin and remove the infection" and "Picking fixes my skin faster than letting it heal"). Sophia was instructed to self-monitor all episodes of checking and skin picking. Next, Sophia made a list of her strategies according to the five categories included in the Comprehensive Model for Behavioral Treatment (ComB; Mansueto et al., 1999): sensory, cognitive, affective, motor, and place/environment (SCAMP).

Sophia struggled, at times, with the definition of BDD as she did not believe scars and acne were "imagined or slight" defects. Acceptance and commitment strategies, including mindfulness exercises were introduced to increase awareness and tolerance for thoughts, emotions, and other triggers for picking. The therapist engaged Sophia in acceptance and commitment therapy (ACT) values clarification exercises to help her reduce time spent on her value on appearance.

As Sophia's urges decreased, the therapist suggested in-session exposure and response prevention exercises to directly practice control of skin picking. A hierarchy of skin picking triggers was constructed, and she was gradually exposed to the triggers and practiced resisting the urges. For example, Sophia was instructed to touch her face and arms until she found a bump that created an urge to pick; she then practiced resisting the urge. Sophia learned that her urges decreased within a short time. It also strengthened her use of various behavioral strategies (e.g., disputing cognitive distortions, using sensory stress balls and other fidget tools).

As Sophia improved on picking and decreased mirror checking by week 3 of treatment, the therapist introduced mirror retraining exercises. Sophia was instructed to practice at home. Although she frequently struggled with neutral language for her skin picking scars, she gradually improved her skills due to her motivation and openness to treatment.

In week 3, exposure and response prevention exercises were introduced to address body parts of concern. Since she had made significant progress reducing skin picking, she chose to target her skin hierarchy first. Sophia began by removing some of her makeup in front of the therapist and gradually engaged with the receptionists at the office and eventually went to department stores without makeup on. She began posting photos of herself on social media with reduced makeup and was able to tolerate some practice professional photography shoots in preparation for her wedding photos. She was extremely worried about breaking out during her honeymoon at a Caribbean beach resort, so she agreed to practice being in the sun and getting sweaty and hot.

Sophia progressed to addressing her body shape concerns more quickly, as these were secondary concerns for her. The therapist helped her practice wearing her wedding gown and taking photographs during home visits. Her fiancé and parents were incorporated in sessions so they could appropriately support her during the wedding day, as well as in the days leading up to it. Sophia was able to get married and enjoy her honeymoon. She continued treatment on a weekly basis to address urges to skin pick, which waxed and waned. She also had some residual discomfort seeing others without makeup. The therapist continued to address these symptoms and reinforce CT skills for maintenance of treatment gains.

6

Further Reading

Claiborn, J., & Pedrick, C. (2002). *The BDD workbook: Overcome body dysmorphic disorder and end body image obsessions*. New Harbinger Publications.
   This self-help manual provides sufferers strategies and worksheets to implement cognitive therapy and exposure and response prevention. The authors also offer helpful exercises and perspective to build a healthier self-esteem and a balanced body image.

Neziroglu, F., Khemlani-Patel, S., & Santos, M. (2012). *Overcoming body dysmorphic disorder: A cognitive behavioral approach to reclaiming your life.* New Harbinger.
   This self-help book provides individuals with BDD and their families with an understanding of the disorder, ways to differentiate between normal appearance concerns and BDD, case examples, and specific cognitive behavior and acceptance and commitment therapy exercises.

Phillips, K. A. (Ed.) (2005). *The broken mirror: Understanding and treating body dysmorphic disorder* (revised and expanded edition). Oxford University Press.
   Dr. Phillips' seminal book provides a comprehensive and straightforward approach to BDD that is equally valuable to mental health professionals, sufferers, and family members. Topics include how to identify the disorder, BDD across the lifespan, etiology, as well as psychological and medication treatment.

Phillips, K. (2017). *Body dysmorphic disorder: Advances in research and clinical practice.* Oxford University Press.
   This edited comprehensive academic book thoroughly covers all aspects of body dysmorphic disorder including phenomenology, cultural and ethic aspects, etiology, pathophysiology, treatment for adolescents and adults, and cosmetic surgery.

Veale, D., & Neziroglu, F. (2010). *Body dysmorphic disorder: A treatment manual.* John Wiley.
   The treatment manual reviews theoretical models of BDD etiology in depth, which provides a framework for the application of psychological treatment techniques. The authors cover assessment, engagement, and multiple practical techniques including exposure therapy, cognitive therapy, as well as lesser-known strategies, such as imagery rescripting and attentional training.

Wilhelm, S., Phillips, K., & Steketee, G. (2012). *Cognitive behavioral therapy for body dysmorphic disorder: A treatment manual.* Guilford Press.
   This clinician treatment manual provides session by session detailed instructions to implement effective CBT techniques. There are helpful instructions on mirror retraining, treatment engagement, and many practical reproducible patient worksheets and handouts.

7

References

Adams, G., Turner, H., & Bucks, R. (2005). The experience of body dissatisfaction in men. *Body Image, 2,* 271–283. https://doi.org/10.1016/j.bodyim.2005.05.004
American Psychiatric Association. (1980). *Diagnostic and statistical manual of mental disorders* (3rd ed.).
American Psychiatric Association. (1987). *Diagnostic and statistical manual of mental disorders* (3rd ed., rev.).
American Psychiatric Association. (2013). *Diagnostic and statistical manual of mental disorders* (5th ed.).
Awad, G. H., Norwood, C., Taylor, D. S., Martinez, M., McClain, S., Jones, B., Holman, A., & Chapman-Hillard, C. (2015). Beauty and body image concerns among African American college women. *Journal of Black Psychology, 41,* 540–564. https://doi.org/10.1177/0095798414550864
Azrin, N. H., & Nunn, R. G. (1973). Habit reversal: A method of eliminating nervous habits and tics. *Behaviour Research and Therapy, 11,* 619–628. https://doi.org/10.1016/0005-7967(73)90119-8
Baldock, E., & Veale, D. (2017). The self as an aesthetic object: Body image, beliefs about the self, and shame in a cognitive model of body dysmorphic disorder. In K. A. Phillips (Ed.), *Body dysmorphic disorder: Advances in research and clinical practice* (pp. 299–310). Oxford University Press.
Bandura, A. (1977). *Social learning theory.* Prentice Hall.
Barr, L. C., Goodman, W. K., & Price, L. H. (1992). Acute exacerbation of body dysmorphic disorder during tryptophan depletion. *American Journal of Psychiatry, 149*(10), 1406–1407. https://doi.org/10.1176/ajp.149.10.1406a
Beck, A. T. (1976). *Cognitive therapy and the emotional disorders*. Penguin.
Beck, A. T., Kovacs, M., & Weissman, A. (1979). Assessment of suicidal intention: The Scale for Suicide Ideation. *Journal of Consulting and Clinical Psychology, 47*(2), 343–352. https://doi.org/10.1037/0022-006X.47.2.343
Bogels, S. M. (2006). Task concentration training versus applied relaxation, in combination with cognitive therapy, for social phobia patients with fear of blushing, trembling, and sweating. *Behavior Research and Therapy, 44,* 1199–1210. https://doi.org/10.1016/j.brat.2005.08.010
Boyda, D., & Shevlin, M. (2011). Childhood victimization as a predictor of muscle dysmorphia in adult male bodybuilders. *Irish Journal of Psychology, 32,* 105–115. https://doi.org/10.1080/03033910.2011.616289
Brawman-Mintzer, O., Lydiard, R., Phillips, K., Morton, A., Czepowica, V., Emmanuel, N., Villareal, G., Johnson, M., & Ballenger, J. (1995). Body dysmorphic disorder in patients with anxiety disorders and major depression: A comorbidity study. *American Journal of Psychiatry, 152,* 1665–1667.
Brown, G. K., Ten Have, T., Henriques, G. R., Xie, S. X., Hollander, J. E., & Beck, A. T. (2005). Cognitive therapy for the prevention of suicide attempts: A randomized control trial. *Journal of the American Medical Association, 294,* 563–570. https://doi.org/10.1001/jama.294.5.563
Brunswick, R. (1928). A supplement to Freud's "History of an infantile neurosis." *International Journal of Psychoanalysis, 9,* 439–476.

Buhlmann, U., Cook, L. M., Fama, J. M., & Wilhelm, S. (2007). Perceived teasing experiences in body dysmorphic disorder. *Body Image, 4,* 381–385. https://doi.org/10.1016/j.bodyim.2007.06.004

Buhlmann, U., Etcoff, N. L., & Wilhelm, S. (2006). Emotion recognition bias for contempt and anger in body dysmorphic disorder. *Journal of Psychiatric Research, 40,* 105–111. https://doi.org/10.1016/j.jpsychires.2005.03.006

Buhlmann, U., Glaesmer, H., Mewes, R., Fama, J. M., Wilhelm, S., Brahler, E., & Rief, W. (2010). Updates on the prevalence of body dysmorphic disorder: A population based survey. *Psychiatry Research, 178,* 171–175. https://doi.org/10.1016/j.psychres.2009.05.002

Buhlmann, U., McNally, R. J., Etcoff, N. L., Tuschen-Caffier, B., & Wilhelm, S. (2004). Emotion recognition deficits in body dysmorphic disorder. *Journal of Psychiatric Research, 38*(2), 201–206. https://doi.org/10.1016/S0022-3956(03)00107-9

Buhlmann, U., McNally, R. J., Wilhelm, S., & Florin, I. (2002). Selective processing of emotional information in body dysmorphic disorder. *Journal of Anxiety Disorders, 16*(3), 289–298. https://doi.org/10.1016/S0887-6185(02)00100-7

Buhlmann, U., & Wilhelm, S. (2004). Cognitive factors in body dysmorphic disorder. *Psychiatric Annals, 34*(12), 922–926. https://doi.org/10.3928/0048-5713-20041201-14

Buhlmann, U., Wilhelm, S., Glaesmer, H., Mewes, R., Brähler, E., & Rief, W. (2011). Perceived appearance-related teasing in body dysmorphic disorder: A population-based survey. *International Journal of Cognitive Therapy, 4*(4), 342–348. https://doi.org/10.1521/ijct.2011.4.4.342

Buhlmann, U., Wilhelm, S., McNally, R. J., Tuschen-Caffier, B., Baer, L., & Jenike, M. A. (2002). Interpretive biases for ambiguous information in body dysmorphic disorder. *CNS spectrums, 7*(6), 435–443. https://doi.org/10.1017/S1092852900017946

Campagna, J. D. A., & Bowsher, B. (2016). Muscle dysmorphia among entry-level military personnel. *Military Medicine, 181,* 494–501. https://doi.org/10.7205/MILMED-D-15-00118

Cansever, A., Uzun, O., Donmez, E., & Ozsahin, A. (2003). The prevalence and clinical features of body dysmorphic disorder in college students: A study in a Turkish sample. *Comprehensive Psychiatry, 44,* 60–64. https://doi.org/10.1053/comp.2003.50010

Cash, T. F., Winstead, B. W. & Janda, L. H. (1986). The great American shape-up: Body-image survey report. *Psychology Today, 20*(4), 30–37.

Cash, T. F. (1997). *The body image workbook: An 8-step program for learning to like your looks.* New Harbinger.

Cash, T. F. (2002). Cognitive behavioral perspectives on body image. In T. F. Cash & T. Pruzinsky (Eds.), *Body image: A handbook of theory, research, and clinical practice.* Guilford Press.

Castle, D. J., Molton, M., Hoffman, K., Preston, N. J., & Phillips, K. A. (2004). Correlates of dysmorphic concern in people seeking cosmetic enhancement. *Australian and New Zealand Journal of Psychiatry, 38,* 439–444. https://doi.org/10.1080/j.1440-1614.2004.01381.x

Clark, D. M., & Wells, A. (1995). The cognitive model of social phobia. In R. Heimberg, M. Liebowitz, D. A. Hope, & F. R. Schneier (Eds.), *Social phobia: Diagnosis, assessment, and treatment* (pp. 69–93). Guilford Press.

Coles, M., Phillips, K., Menard, W., Pagano, M., Fay, C., Weisberg, R., & Stout, R. (2006). Body dysmorphic disorder and social phobia: Cross-sectional and prospective data. *Depression and Anxiety, 23,* 26–33. https://doi.org/10.1002/da.20132

Conrado, L. A. (2009). Body dysmorphic disorder in dermatology: Diagnosis, epidemiology and clinical aspects. *Anais Brasileiros de Dermatologia, 84,* 569–581. https://doi.org/10.1590/S0365-05962009000600002

Craske, M. G., Treanor, M., Conway, C., Zbozinek, T., & Vervliet, B. (2014). Maximizing exposure therapy: An inhibitory learning approach. *Behaviour Research and Therapy, 58,* 10–23. https://doi.org/10.1016/j.brat.2014.04.006

Craven, J., & Rodin, G. (1987). Cyproheptadine dependence associated with an atypical somatoform disorder. *Canadian Journal of Psychiatry, 32,* 143–145. https://doi.org/10.1177/070674378703200211

Crerand, C. E., Sarwer, D. B., Magee, L., Gibbons, L. M., Lowe, M. R., Bartlett, S. P., & Whitaker, L. A. (2004). Rate of body dysmorphic disorder among patients seeking facial cosmetic procedures. *Psychiatric Annals, 34,* 958–965. https://doi.org/10.3928/0048-5713-20041201-19

Conroy, M., Menard, W., Fleming-Ives, K., Modha, P., Cerullo, H., & Phillips, K. A. (2008). Prevalence and clinical characteristics of body dysmorphic disorder in an adult inpatient setting. *General Hospital Psychiatry, 30,* 67–72. https://doi.org/10.1016/j.genhosppsych.2007.09.004

Dahlgren, C. L., Lask, B., Landrø, N., & Rø, Ø. (2014). Developing and evaluating cognitive remediation therapy (CRT) for adolescents with anorexia nervosa: A feasibility study. *Clinical Child Psychology and Psychiatry, 19*(3), 476–487. https://doi.org/10.1177/1359104513489980

Deckersbach, T., Savage, C. R., Phillips, K. A., Wilhelm, S., Buhlmann, U., Rauch, S. L., Baer, L., & Jenike, M. A. (2000). Characteristics of memory dysfunction in body dysmorphic disorder. *Journal of the International Neuropsychological Society, 6*(6), 673–681. https://doi.org/10.1017/S1355617700666055

Dehbaneh, M. A. (2019). Effectiveness of acceptance and commitment therapy in improving interpersonal problems, quality of life, and worry in patients with body dysmorphic disorder. *Electronic Journal of General Medicine, 16*(1), em105. https://doi.org/10.29333/ejgm/93468

de Leon, J., Bott, A., & Simpson, G. M. (1989). Dysmorphophobia: Body dysmorphic disorder or delusional disorder, somatic subtype? *Comprehensive Psychiatry, 30,* 457–472. https://doi.org/10.1016/0010-440X(89)90075-8

Didie, E. R., Menard, W., Stern, A. P., & Phillips, K. A. (2008). Occupational functioning and impairment in adults with body dysmorphic disorder. *Comprehensive Psychiatry, 49,* 561–569. https://doi.org/10.1016/j.comppsych.2008.04.003

Didie, E. R., Tortolani, C. C., Pope, C. G., Menard, W., Fay, C., & Phillips, K. A. (2006). Childhood abuse and neglect in body dysmorphic disorder. *Childhood Abuse and Neglect, 30,* 1105–1115. https://doi.org/10.1016/j.chiabu.2006.03.007

Downing, P. E., Jiang, Y., Shuman, M., & Kanwisher, N. (2001). A cortical area selective for visual processing of the human body. *Science, 293*(5539), 2470–2473.

Dyl, J., Kittler, J., Phillips, K. A., & Hunt, J. I. (2006). Body dysmorphic disorder and other clinically significant body image concerns in adolescent psychiatric inpatients: Prevalence and clinical characteristics. *Child Psychiatry and Human Development, 36,* 369–382. https://doi.org/10.1007/s10578-006-0008-7

Eisen, J. L., Phillips, K. A., Baer, L., Beer, D. A., Atala, K. D., & Rasmussen, S. A. (1998). The Brown Assessment of Beliefs Scale: Reliability and validity. *American Journal of Psychiatry, 155,* 102–108. https://doi.org/10.1176/ajp.155.1.102

Eisen, J. L., Phillips, K. A., Coles, M. E., Rasmussen, S. A. (2004). Insight in obsessive compulsive disorder and body dysmorphic disorder. *Comprehensive Psychiatry, 45,* 10–15. https://doi.org/10.1016/j.comppsych.2003.09.010

Enander, J., Andersson, E., Mataix-Cols, D., Lichtenstein, L., Alström, K., Andersson, G., et al. (2016). Therapist guided internet based cognitive behavioural therapy for body dysmorphic disorder: Single blind randomised controlled trial. *BMJ, 352*(241). https://doi.org/10.1136/bmj.i241

Feusner, J. D., Moller, H., Alstein, L., Sugar, C., Bookheimer, S., Yoon, J., & Hembacher, E. (2010). Inverted face processing in body dysmorphic disorder. *Journal of Psychiatric Research, 44*(15), 1088–1094. https://doi.org/10.1016/j.jpsychires.2010.03.015

Feusner, J. D., Moody, T., Hembacher, E., Townsend, J., McKinley, M., Moller, H., & Bookheimer, S. (2010). Abnormalities of visual processing and frontostriatal systems in body dysmorphic disorder. *Archives of General Psychiatry, 67,* 197–205. https://doi.org/10.1001/archgenpsychiatry.2009.190

Feusner, J. D., Neziroglu, F., Wilhelm, S., Mancusi, L., & Bohon, C. (2010). What causes BDD: Research findings and a proposed model. *Psychiatric Annals, 40,* 349–355. https://doi.org/10.3928/00485713-20100701-08

Feusner, J. D., Phillips, K. A., & Stein, D. J. (2010). Olfactory reference syndrome: Issues for DSM-V. *Depression and Anxiety, 27,* 592–599. https://doi.org/10.1002/da.20688

Feusner, J. D., Townsend, J., Bystritsky, A., & Bookheimer, S. (2007). Visual information processing faces in body dysmorphic disorder. *Archives of General Psychiatry, 64*(12), 1417–1425. https://doi.org/10.1001/archpsyc.64.12.1417

Feusner, J. D., Townsend, J., Bystritsky, A., McKinley, M., Moller, H., & Bookheimer, S. (2009). Regional brain volumes and symptom severity in body dysmorphic disorder. *Psychiatry Research: Neuroimaging, 172*(2), 161–167. https://doi.org/10.1016/j.pscychresns.2008.12.003

First, M. B., Williams, J. B. W., Karg, R. S., & Spitzer, R. L. (2015). *Structured Clinical Interview for DSM-5 – Research Version* (SCID-5 for DSM-5, Research Version; SCID-5-RV). American Psychiatric Association.

Foa, E. B., & Rothbaum, B. O. (1998). *Treating the trauma of rape: Cognitive-behavioral therapy for PTSD.* Guilford Press.

Frare, F., Perugi, G., Ruffolo, G., & Toni, C. (2004). Obsessive compulsive disorder and body dysmorphic disorder: A comparison of clinical features. *European Psychiatry, 19,* 292–298. https://doi.org/10.1016/j.eurpsy.2004.04.014

Frias, A., Palma, C., Farriols, N., & Gonzalez, L. (2015). Comorbidity between obsessive compulsive disorder and body dysmorphic disorder: Prevalence, explanatory theories, and clinical characterization. *Neuropsychiatric Disease and Treatment, 11,* 2233–2244. https://doi.org/10.2147/NDT.S67636

Frontenelle, L. F., Telles, L. L., Nazar, B. P., deMenezes, G. B., Do Nascimento, A. L. (2006). A sociodemographic, phenomenological, and long term follow up study of patients with body dysmorphic disorder in Brazil. *International Journal of Psychiatry in Medicine, 36,* 243–259. https://doi.org/10.2190/B6XM-HLHQ-7X6C-8GC0

Garner, D. (1997). The 1997 body image survey results. *Psychology Today, 30*(1), 30–46.

Gordon, K. H., Castro, Y., Sitnikov, L., & Holm-Denoma, J. M. (2010). Cultural body shape ideals and eating disorder symptoms among White, Latina, and Black college women. *Cultural Diversity and Ethnic Minority Psychology, 16,* 135–143. https://doi.org/10.1037/a0018671

Grant, J. E., Kim, S. W., & Crow, S. J. (2001). Prevalence and clinical features of body dysmorphic disorder in adolescent and adult psychiatric inpatients. *Journal of Clinical Psychiatry, 62,* 517–522. https://doi.org/10.4088/JCP.v62n07a03

Grant, J. E., Menard, & Phillips, K. A. (2006). Pathological skin picking in individuals with body dysmorphic disorder. *General Hospital Psychiatry, 28,* 487–493. https://doi.org/10.1016/j.genhosppsych.2006.08.009

Greenberg, J. L., Weingarden, H., Reuman, L., Abrams, D., Mothi, S. S., & Wilhelm, S. (2018). Set shifting and visuospatial organization deficits in body dysmorphic disorder. *Psychiatry Research, 260,* 182–186. https://doi.org/10.1016/j.psychres.2017.11.062

Gunstad, J., & Phillips, K. A. (2003). Axis I comorbidity in body dysmorphic disorder. *Comprehensive Psychiatry, 44,* 270–276. https://doi.org/10.1016/S0010-440X(03)00088-9

Hanes, K. (1996). Serotonin, psilocybin, and body dysmorphic disorder: A case report. *Journal of Clinical Psychopharmacology, 16,* 188–189. https://doi.org/10.1097/00004714-199604000-00011

Harrison, A., Fernandez de la Cruz, L., Enander, J., Radua, J., Mataix-Cols, D. (2016). Cognitive-behavioral therapy for body dysmorphic disorder: A systematic review and meta-analysis of randomized controlled trials. *Clinical Psychology Review, 48,* 43–51. https://doi.org/10.1016/j.cpr.2016.05.007

Hart, A., & Niemiec, M. (2017). Comorbidity and personality in body dysmorphic disorder. In M. Niemiec (Ed.), *Body dysmorphic disorder: Advances in research and clinical practice* (pp. 125–136). Oxford University Press. https://doi.org/10.1093/med/9780190254131.003.0011

Hart, A. S., & Phillips, K. A. (2013). Symmetry concerns as a symptom of body dysmorphic disorder. *Journal of Obsessive-Compulsive and Related Disorders, 2*(3), 292–298. https://doi.org/10.1016/j.jocrd.2013.04.004

7. References

Hayes, S. C., Strosahl, K. D., & Wilson, K. G. (2011). *Acceptance and commitment therapy: The process and practice of mindful change* (2nd ed.). Guilford Press.

Hayes, S. (2005). *Get out of your mind and into your life: The new acceptance and commitment therapy*. New Harbinger Publications

Heinberg, L. J., Thompson, J. K., & Stormer, S. (1995). Development and validation of the Sociocultural Attitudes Towards Appearance Questionnaire (SATAQ). *International Journal of Eating Disorders, 17,* 81–89. https://doi.org/10.1002/1098-108X(199501)17:1<81::AID-EAT2260170111>3.0.CO;2-Y

Hollander, E., Allen, A., Kwon, J., Aronowitz, B., Schmeidler, J., Wong, & Simeon, D. (1999). Clomipramine vs desipramine crossover trial in body dysmorphic disorder: Selective efficacy of a serotonin reuptake inhibitor in imagined ugliness. *Archives of General Psychiatry, 56,* 1033–1039. https://doi.org/10.1001/archpsyc.56.11.1033

Hollander, E., Kim, S., Khanna, S., & Pallanti, S. (2007). Obsessive compulsive disorder and obsessive compulsive spectrum disorders: Diagnostic and dimensional issues. *CNS Spectrum, 12*(2 Suppl 3), 5–13. https://doi.org/10.1017/S1092852900002467

Hollander, E., & Wong, C. (1995). Introduction: Obsessive compulsive spectrum disorders. *Journal of Clinical Psychiatry, 56,* 3–6.

Ikebuchi, E., Sato, S., Yamaguchi, S., Shimodaira, M., Taneda, A., Hatsuse, N., Watanabe, Y., Sakata, M., Satake, N., Nishio, M., & Ito, J. (2017). Does improvement of cognitive functioning by cognitive remediation therapy effect work outcomes in severe mental illness? A secondary analysis of a randomized controlled trial. *Psychiatry and Clinical Neurosciences, 71*(5), 301–308.

Ipser, J. C., Sander, C., & Stein, D. J. (2009). Pharmacotherapy and psychotherapy for body dysmorphic disorder. *Cochrane Database of Systematic Reviews, 1,* CD005332. https://doi.org/10.1002%2F14651858.CD005332.pub2

Jobes, D. A. (2012). The collaborative assessment and management of suicidality (CAMS): An evolving evidence based clinical approach to suicidal risk. *Suicide and Life-Threatening Behavior, 42,* 640–653. https://doi.org/10.1111/j.1943-278X.2012.00119.x

Jobes, D. A., Au, J. S., & Siegelman, A. (2015). Psychological approaches to suicide treatment and prevention. *Current Treatment Options in Psychiatry, 2,* 363–370. https://doi.org/10.1007/s40501-015-0064-3

Kacar, A. D., Ozuguz, P., Bagcioglu, E., Coskun, K. S., Uzel Tas, H., Polat, S., & Karaca, S. (2014). The frequency of body dysmorphic disorder in dermatology and cosmetic dermatology clinics: A study from Turkey. *Clinical and Experimental Dermatology, 39,* 433–438. https://doi.org/10.1111/ced.12304

Kerwin, L., Hovav, S., Hellemann, G., & Feusner, J. (2014). Impairment in local and global processing and set shifting in body dysmorphic disorder. *Journal of Psychiatric Research, 57,* 41–50. https://doi.org/10.1016/j.jpsychires.2014.06.003

Khemlani-Patel, S. (2001). Cognitive and behavior therapy for body dysmorphic disorder: A comparative investigation. [Doctoral dissertation, Hofstra University]. *Dissertation Abstracts International: Section B: The Sciences and Engineering, 62,* 1087.

Khemlani-Patel, S., Neziroglu, F., & Mancusi, L. M. (2011). Cognitive-behavioral therapy for body dysmorphic disorder: A comparative investigation. *International Journal of Cognitive Therapy, 4,* 363–380. https://doi.org/10.1521/ijct.2011.4.4.363

Koran, L. M., Abujaoude, E., Large, M. D., & Serpe, R. T. (2008). The prevalence of body dysmorphic disorder in the United States adult population. *CNS Spectrums, 13,* 316–322. https://doi.org/10.1017/S1092852900016436

Lambrou, C., Veale, D., & Wilson, G. D. (2011). The role of aesthetic sensitivity in body dysmorphic disorder. *Journal of Abnormal Psychology, 120,* 443–453. https://doi.org/10.1037/a0022300

Levine, M. P., & Smolak, L. (2002). Body image development in adolescence. In T. F. Cash & T. Pruzinsky (Eds.), *Body image: A handbook of theory, research, and clinical practice* (pp. 74–82). Guilford Press.

Linde, J., Ruck, C., Bjureberg, J., Ivanov, V. Z., Djurfeldt, D. R., & Ramnero, J. (2015). Acceptance-based exposure therapy for body dysmorphic disorder: A pilot study. *Behavior Therapy, 46,* 423–431. https://doi.org/10.1016/j.beth.2015.05.002

Linehan, M. (1993). *Cognitive behavioral treatment of borderline personality disorder.* Guilford Press.

Lipkens, G., Hayes, S. C., & Hayes, L. J. (1993). Longitudinal study of derived stimulus relations in an infant. *Journal of the Experimental Analysis of Behavior, 56,* 201–239.

Madsen, S. K., Bohon, C., & Feusner, J. D. (2013). Visual processing in anorexia nervosa and body dysmorphic disorder: Similarities, differences, and future research directions. *Journal of Psychiatric Research, 47,* 1483–1491. https://doi.org/10.1016/j.jpsychires.2013.06.003

Mansueto, C. S., Golomb, R. G., & Thomas, A. M. (1999). A comprehensive model for behavioral treatment of trichotillomania. *Cognitive and Behavioral Practice, 6,* 23–43. https://doi.org/10.1016/S1077-7229(99)80038-8

Mausbach, B. T., Moore, R., Roesch, S., Cardenas, V., & Patterson, T. L. (2010). The relationship between homework compliance and therapy outcomes: An updated meta-analysis. *Cognitive Therapy Research, 34,* 429–438. https://doi.org/10.1007/s10608-010-9297-z

McCabe, M. P., & Ricciardelli, L. A. (2004). Body image dissatisfaction among males across the lifespan: A review of past literature. *Journal of Psychosomatic Research, 56,* 675–685. https://doi.org/10.1016/S0022-3999(03)00129-6

McConnaughy, E. A., Prochaska, J. O., & Velicer, W. F. (1983). Stages of change in psychotherapy: Measurement and sample profiles. *Psychotherapy: Theory, Research and Practice, 20*(3), 368–375. https://doi.org/10.1037/h0090198

McCurdy-McKinnon, D., & Feusner, J. (2017). Neurobiology of body dysmorphic disorder: Heritability/genetics, brain circuitry, and visual processing. In K. Phillips (Ed.), *Body dysmorphic disorder: Advances in research and clinical practice* (pp. 253–276). Oxford University Press.

McKay, D. (1999). Two year follow up of behavioral treatment and maintenance for body dysmorphic disorder. *Behavior Modification, 23*(4), 620–629. https://doi.org/10.1177/0145445599234006

McKay, D., Neziroglu, F., & Yaryura-Tobias, J. A. (1997). Comparison of clinical characteristics in obsessive-compulsive disorder and body dysmorphic disorder. *Journal of Anxiety Disorders, 11,* 447–454. https://doi.org/10.1016/S0887-6185(97)00020-0

McKay, D., Todaro, J., & Neziroglu, F. (1997). Body dysmorphic disorder: A preliminary evaluation of treatment and maintenance using exposure with response prevention. *Behavior Research and Therapy, 35*(1), 67–70. https://doi.org/10.1016/S0005-7967(96)00082-4

McKenna, P. J. (1984). Disorders with overvalued ideas. *British Journal of Psychiatry, 145,* 579–585. https://doi.org/10.1192/bjp.145.6.579

Miller, W. R., & Rollnick, S. (1991). *Motivational interviewing: Preparing people to change addictive behavior.* Guilford Press.

Miller, W. R., & Rollnick, S. (2012). *Motivational interviewing: Helping people change.* Guilford Press.

Morselli, E. (1891). Sulla dismorfofobia e sulla tafefobia [On dysmorphophobia and taphephobia]. *Bolletinno della R Accademia di Genova, 6,* 110–119.

Neziroglu, F. (2004). *How to apply cognitive and behavior therapy for body dysmorphic disorder* [Paper presentation]. Symposium on body dysmorphic disorder, meeting of the American Psychiatric Association, New York, NY, USA.

Neziroglu, F., Borda, T., Khemlani-Patel, S., & Bonasera, B. (2018). Prevalence of bullying in a pediatric sample of body dysmorphic disorder. *Comprehensive Psychiatry, 87,* 12–16. https://doi.org/10.1016/j.comppsych.2018.08.014

Neziroglu, F., Khemlani-Patel, S., & Jacofsky, M. (2009). Body dysmorphic disorder: Symptoms, models, and treatment interventions. In G. Simos (Ed.), *Cognitive behaviour therapy: A guide for the practising clinician* (Vol. 2). Routledge.

Neziroglu, F., Khemlani-Patel, S., & Veale, D. (2008). Social learning theory and cognitive behavioral models of body dysmorphic disorder. *Body Image, 5*(1), 28–38. https://doi.org/10.1016/j.bodyim.2008.01.002

Neziroglu, F., Khemlani-Patel, S., & Yaryura-Tobias, J. A. (2006). Rates of abuse in body dysmorphic disorder and obsessive compulsive disorder. *Body Image, 3*(2), 189–193. https://doi.org/10.1016/j.bodyim.2006.03.001

Neziroglu, F., McKay, D., Todaro, J., & Yaryura-Tobias, J. A. (1996). Effect of cognitive behavior therapy on persons with body dysmorphic disorder and comorbid Axis II diagnoses. *Behavior Therapy, 27*(1), 67–77. https://doi.org/10.1016/S0005-7894(96)80036-0

Neziroglu, F., McKay, D., Yaryura-Tobias, J. A., Stevens, K. P., & Todaro, J. (1999). The Overvalued Ideas Scale: Development, reliability, and validity in obsessive compulsive disorder. *Behavior Research and Therapy, 37,* 881–902. https://doi.org/10.1016/S0005-7967(98)00191-0

Neziroglu, F., Roberts, M., & Yaryura-Tobias, J. A. (2004). A behavioral model for body dysmorphic disorder. *Psychiatric Annals, 34,* 915–920. https://doi.org/10.3928/0048-5713-20041201-13

Neziroglu F., & Yaryura-Tobias, J. A. (1993). Body dysmorphic disorder: Phenomenology and case descriptions. *Behavior Psychotherapy, 21,* 27–36. https://doi.org/10.1017/S0141347300017778

Niedenthal, P. M., & Wood, A. (2019). Does emotion influence visual perception? Depends on how you look at it. *Cognition Emotion, 33,* 77–84. https://doi.org/10.1080/02699931.2018.1561424

Osman, S., Cooper, M., Hackman, A., & Veale, D. (2004). Spontaneously occurring images and early memories in people with body dysmorphic disorder. *Memory, 12*(4), 428–436. https://doi.org/10.1080/09658210444000043

Peelen, M. V., & Downing, P. E. (2005). Selectivity for the human body in the fusiform gyrus. *Journal of Neurophysiology, 93*(1), 603–608. https://doi.org/10.1152/jn.00513.2004

Perugi, G., Akiskal, H. S., Giannotti, D., Frare, F., DiVaio, S., & Cassano, G. B. (1997). Gender related differences in body dysmorphic disorder. *Journal of Nervous and Mental Disease, 185,* 578–582. https://doi.org/10.1097/00005053-199709000-00007

Perugi, G., Giannotti, D., Di Vaio, S., Frare, F., Saettoni, M., & Cassano, G. B. (1996). Fluvoxamine in treatment of body dysmorphic disorder (dysmorphophobia). *International Clinical Psychopharmacology, 11,* 247–254. https://doi.org/10.1097/00004850-199612000-00006

Phillips, K. A. (2000). Quality of life for patients with body dysmorphic disorder. *Journal of Nervous and Mental Disease, 188,* 170–175. https://doi.org/10.1097/00005053-200003000-00007

Phillips, K. A. (2004). Psychosis in body dysmorphic disorder. *Journal of Psychiatric Research, 38,* 63–72. https://doi.org/10.1016/S0022-3956(03)00098-0

Phillips, K. A. (2005). *The broken mirror: Understanding and treating body dysmorphic disorder* (Revised & exp. ed.). Oxford University Press.

Phillips, K. A. (2010). Pharmacotherapy for body dysmorphic disorder. *Psychiatric Annals, 40*(7), 325–332. https://doi.org/10.3928/00485713-20100701-05

Phillips, K. A., Albertini, R. S., & Rasmussen, S. A. (2002). A randomized placebo-controlled trial of fluoxetine in body dysmorphic disorder. *Archives of General Psychiatry, 9,* 381–388. https://doi.org/10.1001/archpsyc.59.4.381

Phillips, K. A., Atala, K. D., & Pope, H. G. (1995). *Diagnostic instruments for body dysmorphic disorder.* New Research Program and Abstracts. American Psychiatric Association 148th annual meeting, Miami, FL, United States.

Phillips, K. A., Coles, M. E., Menard, W., Yen, S., Fay, C., & Weisberg, R. B. (2005). Suicidal ideation and suicide attempts in body dysmorphic disorder. *Journal of Clinical Psychiatry, 66*(6), 717–725. https://doi.org/10.4088/JCP.v66n0607

Phillips, K. A., & Diaz, S. F. (1997). Gender differences in body dysmorphic disorder. *Journal of Nervous and Mental Disease, 185,* 570–577. https://doi.org/10.1097/00005053-199709000-00006

Phillips, K. A., Didie, E. R., & Menard, W. (2007). Clinical features and correlates of major depressive disorder in individuals with body dysmorphic disorder. *Journal of Affective Disorders, 97,* 129–135. https://doi.org/10.1016/j.jad.2006.06.006

Phillips, K. A., Didie, E. R., Menard, W., Pagano, M. E., Fay, C., & Weisberg, R. B. (2006). Clinical features of body dysmorphic disorder in adolescents and adults. *Psychiatry Research, 141*(3), 305–314.

Phillips, K. A., Dufresne, R. G., Jr., Wilkel, C. S., & Vittorio, C. C. (2000). Rate of body dysmorphic disorder in dermatology patients. *Journal of American Academy of Dermatology, 42,* 436–441. https://doi.org/10.1016/S0190-9622(00)90215-9

Phillips, K. A., Dwight, M. M., McElroy, S. L. (1998). Efficacy and safety of fluvoxamine in body dysmorphic disorder. *Journal of Clinical Psychiatry, 59,* 165–171. https://doi.org/10.4088/JCP.v59n0404

Phillips, K. A., Hollander, E., Rasmussen, S. A., Aronowitz, B. R., DeCaria, C., & Goodman, W. K. (1997). A severity rating scale for body dysmorphic disorder: Development, reliability, and validity of a modified version of the Yale-Brown Obsessive Compulsive Scale. *Psychopharmacology Bulletin, 33,* 17–22.

Phillips, K. A., Keshaviah, A., Dougherty, D., Stout, R. L., Menard, W., & Wilhelm, S. (2016). Pharmacotherapy relapse prevention in body dysmorphic disorder: A double-blind placebo-controlled trial. *American Journal of Psychiatry, 173,* 887–895. https://doi.org/10.1176/appi.ajp.2016.15091243

Phillips, K. A., & McElroy, S. (2000). Personality disorders and traits in patients with body dysmorphic disorder. *Comprehensive Psychiatry, 41*(4), 229–236.

Phillips, K. A., McElroy, S. L., Keck, P. E., Pope, H. G., & Hudson, J. I. (1994). A comparison of delusional and nondelusional body dysmorphic disorder in 100 cases. *Psychopharmacology Bulletin, 30,* 179–186.

Phillips, K. A., & Menard, W. (2006). Suicidality in body dysmorphic disorder: A prospective study. *American Journal of Psychiatry, 163,* 1280–1282. https://doi.org/10.1176/ajp.2006.163.7.1280

Phillips, K. A., Menard, W., Fay, C., & Weisberg, R. (2005). Demographic characteristics, phenomenology, comorbidity, and family history in 200 individuals with body dysmorphic disorder. *Psychosomatics, 46,* 3170325. https://doi.org/10.1176/appi.psy.46.4.317

Phillips, K. A., Menard, W., Quinn, E., & Didie, E. R. (2013). A 4-year prospective observational follow-up study of course and predictors of course in body dysmorphic disorder. *Psychological Medicine, 43*(5), 1109–1117. https://doi.org/10.1017/S0033291712001730

Phillips, K., & Najjar, F. (2003). An open label study of citalopram in body dysmorphic disorder. *Journal of Clinical Psychiatry, 64,* 715–720. https://doi.org/10.4088/JCP.v64n0615

Phillips, K. A., Pagano, M. E., Menard, W., Fay, C., & Stout, R. L. (2005). Predictors of remission from body dysmorphic disorder: A prospective study. *Journal of Nervous and Mental Disease, 193,* 564–567. https://doi.org/10.1097/01.nmd.0000172681.51661.54

Phillips, K. A., Pagano, M. E., Menard, W., & Stout, R. L. (2006). A 12-month follow-up study of the course of body dysmorphic disorder. *American Journal of Psychiatry, 163*(5), 907–912. https://doi.org/10.1176/ajp.2006.163.5.907

Phillips, K. A., Pinto, A., Hart, A. S., Coles, M. E., Eisen, J. L., Menard, W., & Rasmussen, S. A. (2012). A comparison of insight in body dysmorphic disorder and obsessive compulsive disorder. *Journal of Psychiatry Research, 46,* 1293–1299. https://doi.org/10.1016/j.jpsychires.2012.05.016

Phillips, K. A., & Rasmussen, S. A. (2004). Change in psychosocial functioning and quality of life of patients with body dysmorphic disorder. *Psychosomatics, 45,* 438–444. https://doi.org/10.1176/appi.psy.45.5.438

Prazeres, A. M., Nascimento, A. L., & Fontenelle, L. F. (2013). Cognitive behavioral therapy for body dysmorphic disorder: A review of its efficacy. *Neuropsychiatric Disease and Treatment, 9,* 307–316.

Pryse-Phillips, W. (1971). An olfactory reference syndrome. *Acta Psychiatrica Scandinavica, 47,* 484–509. https://doi.org/10.1111/j.1600-0447.1971.tb03705.x

Resick, P. A., Monson, C. M., & Chard, M. (2016). *Cognitive processing therapy for PTSD: A comprehensive manual.* Guilford Press.

Rief, W., Buhlmann, U., Wilhelm, S., Borkenhagen, A., & Brahler, E. (2006). The prevalence of body dysmorphic disorders: A population based survey. *Psychological Medicine, 36*(6), 877–885. https://doi.org/10.1017/S0033291706007264

Rieves, L., & Cash, T. F. (1996). Social developmental factors and women's body-image attitudes. *Journal of Social Behavior and Personality, 11,* 63–78.

Ritter, V., & Stangier, U. (2015). Seeing in the mind's eye: Imagery rescripting for patients with body dysmorphic disorder: A single case series. *Journal of Behavior Therapy and Experimental Psychiatry, 50,* 187–195.

Rosen, J. C., & Ramirez, E. (1998). A comparison of eating disorders and body dysmorphic disorder on body image and psychological adjustment. *Journal of Psychosomatic Research, 44,* 441–449. https://doi.org/10.1016/S0022-3999(97)00269-9

Rosen, J. C., & Reiter, J. (1996). Development of the body dysmorphic disorder examination. *Behavior Research and Therapy, 34,* 755–766. https://doi.org/10.1016/0005-7967(96)00024-1

Rosen, J. C., Reiter, J., & Orosan, P. (1995). Cognitive-behavioral body image therapy for body dysmorphic disorder. *Journal of Consulting and Clinical Psychology, 63,* 263–9. https://doi.org/10.1037/0022-006X.63.2.263

Ruffolo, J. S., Phillips, K. A., Menard, W., Fay, C., & Weisberg, R. B. (2006). Comorbidity of body dysmorphic disorder and eating disorders: Severity of psychopathology and body image disturbance. *International Journal of Eating Disorders, 39,* 11–19. https://doi.org/10.1002/eat.20219

Savage, C., Baer, L., Keuthen, N., Brown, H., Rauch, S., & Jenike, M. (1999). Organizational strategies mediate nonverbal memory impairment in obsessive-compulsive disorder. *Biological Psychiatry, 45*(7), 905–916. https://doi.org/10.1016/S0006-3223(98)00278-9

Schwarzlose, R. F., Baker, C. I., & Kanwisher, N. (2005). Separate face and body selectivity on the fusiform gyrus. *Journal of Neuroscience, 25,* 11055–11059. https://doi.org/10.1523/JNEUROSCI.2621-05.2005

Sheehan, D. V., Giddens, J. M., & Sheehan, I. S. (2014). Status update on the Sheehan-Suicidality Tracking Scale (S-STS). *Innovations in Clinical Neuroscience, 11,* 93–140.

Sidali, D. M. (2018). *Assessment of accuracy in detecting distortions in self-referent and neutral photographs in BDD.* Hofstra University.

Smucker, M. R., Dancu, C., Foa, E. B., & Niederee, J. L. (1995). Imagery rescripting: A new treatment for survivors of childhood sexual abuse suffering from posttraumatic stress. *Journal of Cognitive Psychotherapy, 9*(1), 3–17. https://doi.org/10.1891/0889-8391.9.1.3

Spiridon, M., Fischl, B., & Kanwisher, N. (2006). Location and spatial profile of category specific regions in human extrastriate cortex. *Human Brain Mapping, 27*(1), 77–89. https://doi.org/10.1002/hbm.20169

Stormer, S. M., & Thompson, J. E. (1996). Explanations of body image disturbance: A test of maturational status, negative verbal commentary, social comparison, and sociocultural hypotheses. *International Journal of Eating Disorders, 19,* 193–202. https://doi.org/10.1002/(SICI)1098-108X(199603)19:2<193::AID-EAT10>3.0.CO;2-W

Taqui, A. M. et al. (2008). Body dysmorphic disorder: Gender differences and prevalence in a Pakistani medical student population. *BMC Psychiatry, 8,* 8–20. https://doi.org/10.1186/1471-244X-8-20

Taylor, J. C., Wiggett, A. J., & Downing, P. E. (2007). Functional MRI analysis of body and body part representations in the extrastriate and fusiform body areas. *Journal of Neurophysiology, 98*(3), 1626–1633. https://doi.org/10.1152/jn.00012.2007

Tchanturia, K., Davies, H., Roberts, M., Harrison, A., Nakazato, M., Schmidt, U., Treasure, J., & Morris, R. (2012). Poor cognitive flexibility in eating disorders: Examining the evidence using the Wisconsin Card Sorting Task. *PLoS ONE, 7*(1). https://doi.org/10.1371/journal.pone.0028331

Tiggemann, M. (2004). Body image across the adult life span: Stability and change. *Body Image, 1*(1), 29–41. https://doi.org/10.1016/S1740-1445(03)00002-0

Tolin, D. F., Hannan, S., Maltby, N., Diefenbach, G. J., Worhunsky, P., & Brady, R. E. (2007). A randomized controlled trial of self-directed versus therapist-directed cognitive-behavioral therapy for obsessive compulsive disorder patients with prior medication trials. *Behavior Therapy, 38,* 179–191. https://doi.org/10.1016/j.beth.2006.07.001

Van Noppen, B., Steketee, G., McCorkle, B. H., & Pato, M. (1997). Group and multifamily behavioral treatment for obsessive compulsive disorder: A pilot study. *Journal of Anxiety Disorders, 11,* 431–460. https://doi.org/10.1016/S0887-6185(97)00021-2

Van Passel, B., Danner, U., Dingemans, A., van Furth, E., Sternheim, L., van Elburg, A., van Minnen, A., van den Hout, M., Hendriks, G., & Cath, D. (2016). Cognitive remediation therapy (CRT) as a treatment enhancer of eating disorders and obsessive-compulsive disorders: Study protocol for a randomized controlled trial. *BMC Psychiatry, 16*(1), 393.

Veale, D. (2000). Outcome of cosmetic surgery and "DIY" surgery in patients with body dysmorphic disorder. *Psychiatric Bulletin, 24*(6), 218–220.

Veale, D. (2004). Advances in a cognitive behavioural model of body dysmorphic disorder. *Body Image, 1*(1), 113–125.

Veale, D. (2010). Cognitive behavioral therapy for body dysmorphic disorder. *Psychiatric Annals, 40*(7), 333–340. https://doi.org/10.3928/00485713-20100701-06

Veale, D., Anson, M., Miles, S., Pieta, M., Costa, A., & Ellison, N. (2014). Efficacy of cognitive behavior therapy versus anxiety management for body dysmorphic disorder: A randomized controlled trial. *Psychotherapy Psychosomatics, 83*(6), 341–353. https://doi.org/10.1159/000360740

Veale, D., Boocock, A., Gournay, K., Dryden, W., Shah, F., Wilson, R., & Walurn, J. (1996). Body dysmorphic disorder: A survey of fifty cases. *British Journal of Psychiatry, 169,* 196–201. https://doi.org/10.1192/bjp.169.2.196

Veale, D., & Neziroglu, F. (2010). *Body dysmorphic disorder: A treatment manual.* John Wiley.

Vitiello, B., & de Leon, J. (1990). Dysmorphophobia misdiagnosed as obsessive-compulsive disorder. *Psychosomatics, 31*(2), 220–222. https://doi.org/10.1016/S0033-3182(90)72200-1

Vita, A., Deste, G., Barlati, S., Poli, R., Cacciani, P., Peri, L. D., & Sacchetti, E. (2016). Feasibility and effectiveness of cognitive remediation in the treatment of borderline personality disorder. *Neuropsychological Rehabilitation, 28*(3), 416–428. https://doi.org/10.1080/09602011.2016.1148054

Weiner, K. S., & Grill-Spector, K. (2010). Sparsely-distributed organization of face and limb activations in human ventral temporal cortex. *Neuroimage, 52*(4), 1559–1573. https://doi.org/10.1016/j.neuroimage.2010.04.262

Weingarden, H., Curley, E. E., Renshaw, K. D., & Wilhelm, S. (2017). Patient-identified events implicated in the development of body dysmorphic disorder. *Body Image, 21,* 19–25. https://doi.org/10.1016/j.bodyim.2017.02.003

Weingarden, H., & Renshaw, K. (2016). Body dysmorphic symptoms, functional impairment, and depression. The role of appearance-based teasing. *Journal of Psychology, 150*(1), 119–131.

Weingarden, H., Renshaw, K. D., Wilhelm, S., Tangney, J. P., & DiMauro, J. (2016). Anxiety and shame as risk factors for depression, suicidality, and functional impairment in body dysmorphic disorder and obsessive compulsive disorder. *Journal of Nervous and Mental Disease, 204*(11), 832–839. https://doi.org/10.1097/NMD.0000000000000498

Wells, A. (1990). Panic disorder in association with relaxation induced anxiety: An attentional training approach in treatment. *Behavior Therapy, 21,* 273–280. https://doi.org/10.1016/S0005-7894(05)80330-2

Wilhelm, S., Greenberg, J. L., Rosenfield, E., Kasarskis, I., & Blashill, A. J. (2016). The body dysmorphic disorder symptom scale: Development and preliminary validation of a self-report scale of symptom specific dysfunction. *Body Image, 17,* 82–87. https://doi.org/10.1016/j.bodyim.2016.02.006

Wilhelm, S., Otto, M. W., Lohr, B., & Deckersbach, T. (1999). Cognitive behavior group therapy for body dysmorphic disorder: A case series. *Behaviour Research and Therapy, 37,* 71–75. https://doi.org/10.1016/S0005-7967(98)00109-0

Wilhelm, S., Phillips, K. A., Didie, E., Buhlmann, U., Greenberg, J. L., Fama, J. M., Keshaviah, A., & Steketee, G. (2014). Modular cognitive-behavioral therapy for body dysmorphic disorder: A randomized controlled trial. *Behavior Therapy, 45*(3), 314–327. https://doi.org/10.1016/j.beth.2013.12.007

Wilhelm, S., Phillips, K. A., & Steketee, G. (2012). *Cognitive behavioral therapy for body dysmorphic disorder: A treatment manual.* Guildford Press.

Wilhelm, S., Phillips, K., & Steketee, G. (2013). *Cognitive behavioral therapy for body dysmorphic disorder: A treatment manual*. Guilford Press.

Williams, J., Hadjistavropoulos, T., & Sharpe, D. (2006). A meta-analysis of psychological and pharmacological treatments for body dysmorphic disorder. *Behavior Research Therapy, 44*(1), 99–111. https://doi.org/10.1016/j.brat.2004.12.006

Wilson, R., Veale, D., & Freeston, M. (2016). Imagery rescripting for body dysmorphic disorder: A multiple baseline single case experimental design. *Behavior Therapy, 47,* 248–261. https://doi.org/10.1016/j.beth.2015.08.006

Zimmerman, M., & Mattia, J. I. (1999). Differences between clinical and research practices in diagnosing borderline personality disorder. *American Journal of Psychiatry, 156*(10), 1570–1574. https://doi.org/10.1176/ajp.156.10.1570

8

Appendix: Tools and Resources

The materials reproduced on the following pages can also be downloaded free of charge from the Hogrefe website after registration.

Appendix 1:   Attractiveness Bell Curve
Appendix 2:   Early Influences on BDD Development
Appendix 3:   My BDD Model
Appendix 4:   Cognitive Distortions
Appendix 5:   Cognitive Therapy Thought Record
Appendix 6:   Values
Appendix 7:   Compulsive, Safety-Seeking, and Avoidance Behaviors
Appendix 8:   Exposure Hierarchy
Appendix 9:   Holistic Perceptual Retraining
Appendix 10: Maintenance and Relapse Prevention Plan

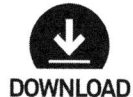
DOWNLOAD

How to proceed:

1. Create a user account (or, if you have already one, please log in)

For customers from the USA, Canada, and the rest of the world:
hgf.io/login-us

For European customers:
hgf.io/login-eu

2. Download your supplementary materials

Go to **My supplementary materials** in your account dashboard and enter the code below. You will automatically be redirected to the download area, where you can access and download the supplementary materials.

Code: B-0B1BOZ

To make sure you have permanent direct access to all the materials, we recommend that you download them and save them on your computer.

Attractiveness Bell Curve

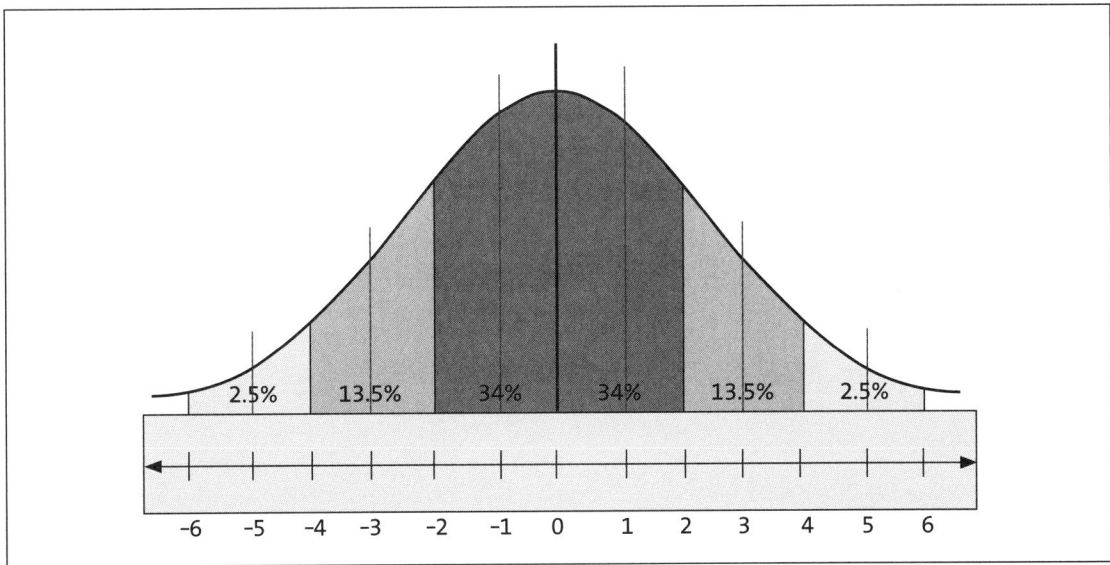

Description

A *bell curve* is a statistical graph that demonstrates the normal distribution in many situations including psychology and business. The middle line represents the average (mean) score. And as you move away from the middle, there is a smaller and smaller percentage of people who fall into those ranges.

For example, if we measured the height of 100 women, 68% would fall within the average range. The percentage of women who are taller is to the right of the average range, while the percentage of women who are shorter is represented to the left of the average range.

Let us now consider measuring attractiveness in the same way. Imagine that a majority of the population would fall into the average range of attractiveness, with the percentage of the population getting progressively more attractive to the right of the average range and less attractive to the left of the average range.

Instructions

Using the graph above, please answer the following questions regarding your opinion of your attractiveness.

Overall Appearance

A. Choose a number to represent how you currently rate your overall attractiveness as compared with the general population. _____

B. Choose a number to represent how you would *like* your overall attractiveness to be as compared with the general population (your desired attractiveness). _____

Specific Body Parts

Next, list your top three body parts of concern in order of importance.

1. _____ (Primary body part)
2. _____
3. _____

Primary Body Part of Concern

A. Choose a number to represent how you currently rate your primary body part of concern as compared with the general population. _____

B. Choose a number to represent how you would *like* your primary body part of concern to be as compared with the general population (your desired appearance). _____

Second Body Part of Concern

A. Choose a number to represent how you currently rate your second body part of concern as compared with the general population. _____

B. Choose a number to represent how you would *like* your second body part of concern to be as compared with the general population (your desired appearance). _____

Third Body Part of Concern

A. Choose a number to represent how you currently rate your third body part of concern as compared with the general population. _____

B. Choose a number to represent how you would *like* your third body part of concern to be as compared with the general population (your desired appearance). _____

What percentage of the population do you believe is more attractive than you (0–100%)? _____

Early Influences on BDD Development

Biological Predispostion – List family history of body dysmorphic disorder (BDD), obsessive-compulsive disorder (OCD), depression, or other mental health conditions or significant medical history, such as excessive illnesses, viruses, strep throat:

_____

_____

_____

_____

Childhood Events – Events that contributed to my focus and value on appearance. Parental, cultural messages including media, immediate social experiences such as high school climate, other personal experiences, bullying, trauma, or abuse.

Parental and/or Family Messages (including from siblings, extended family)

_____

_____

_____

_____

Cultural Messages (media, social)

_____

_____

_____

_____

My Immediate Social Environment (school, work, friends, peer influence)

_____

_____

_____

_____

Bullying (If yes, what were you bullied about and at what age?)

_____

_____

_____

_____

Teasing

_____

_____

_____

_____

Rosacia, Acne, Early or Late Puberty

_____

_____

_____

_____

Trauma or Loss

_____

_____

_____

_____

_____

Other Influences (involvement in sports, dance, injury, accidents, etc.)

_____

_____

_____

_____

_____

My BDD Model

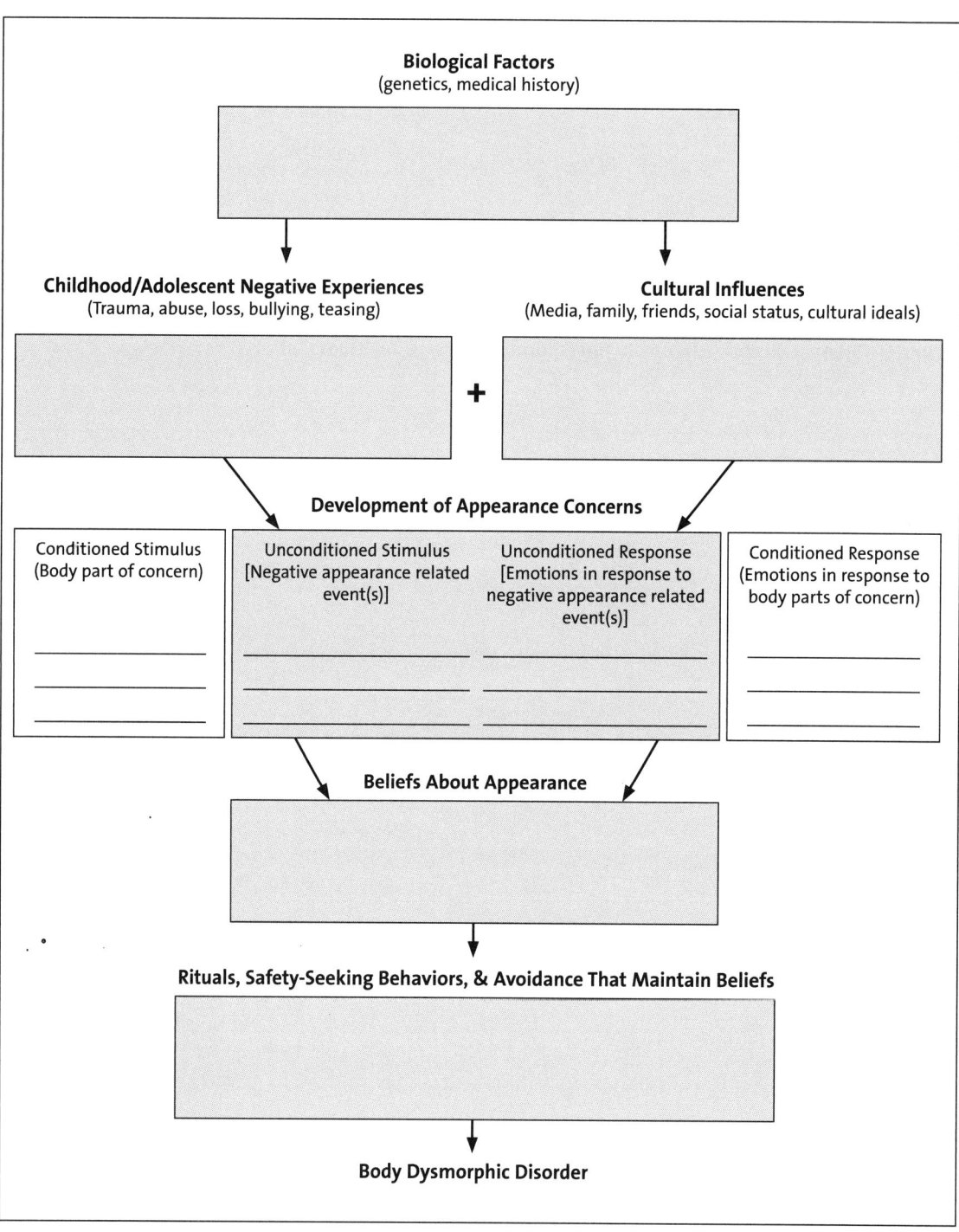

Cognitive Distortions

1. **All or nothing thinking / Black-and-white thinking:** The belief that things are either all or nothing, and there is no middle ground. Seeing things as extremes.
   "If I'm not perfect, then I'm hideous looking."

2. **Catastrophizing:** Exaggerating the meaning or likelihood of things.
   "I will never meet anyone who finds me attractive."

3. **Overgeneralization:** Reaching a general conclusion based on single events or experiences.
   "No one spoke to me at the party; I am boring and unattractive."
   "I am a loser."

4. **Jumping to Conclusions:** Believing one knows what someone is thinking or feeling or what the future holds, without evidence or observations to support it.
   "They were laughing and looking at me, and I am sure it was about my forehead."

   a. **Fortune Telling:** Believing one knows future outcomes. Mistaking predictions as facts about the future.
   "I will never find anyone that I'm attracted to who will also find me attractive."

   b. **Mind Reading:** Believing one knows what someone is thinking or feeling.
   "The girl I was speaking to stopped talking to me, she obviously thinks I'm ugly."
   "The cashier attended to the more attractive girl in line before me because she values attractive people."

5. **Emotional Reasoning:** Believing that the way one feels reflects the reality of events. I feel it therefore it's true.
   "I feel I am unattractive and people don't like me, so this must be true."

6. **Should Statements:** Expressing rigid expectations regarding how oneself or others should behave. Words used include "should, ought, must."
   "I should not have any bumps on my skin."

7. **Mental Filter:** Noticing only the negative aspects of a situation or oneself while ignoring the positive. Selectively attending to certain aspects of an experience.
   "There were only skinny, perfect looking people at the beach. I was the only one with messy hair and overweight."

8. **Disqualifying the Positive:** Rejects positive experiences or feedback as meaningless, disingenuous, or a result of luck.
   "My friend only complimented my hair and outfit that day because they want a ride to school from me." or "Of course my mother complimented my hair, she is my mother and that is what mothers do."

9. **Personalizing:** Misinterpreting someone else's behavior as a reaction to you.
   "The grocery clerk ignored me on purpose and served the more attractive customer."

Cognitive Therapy Thought Record

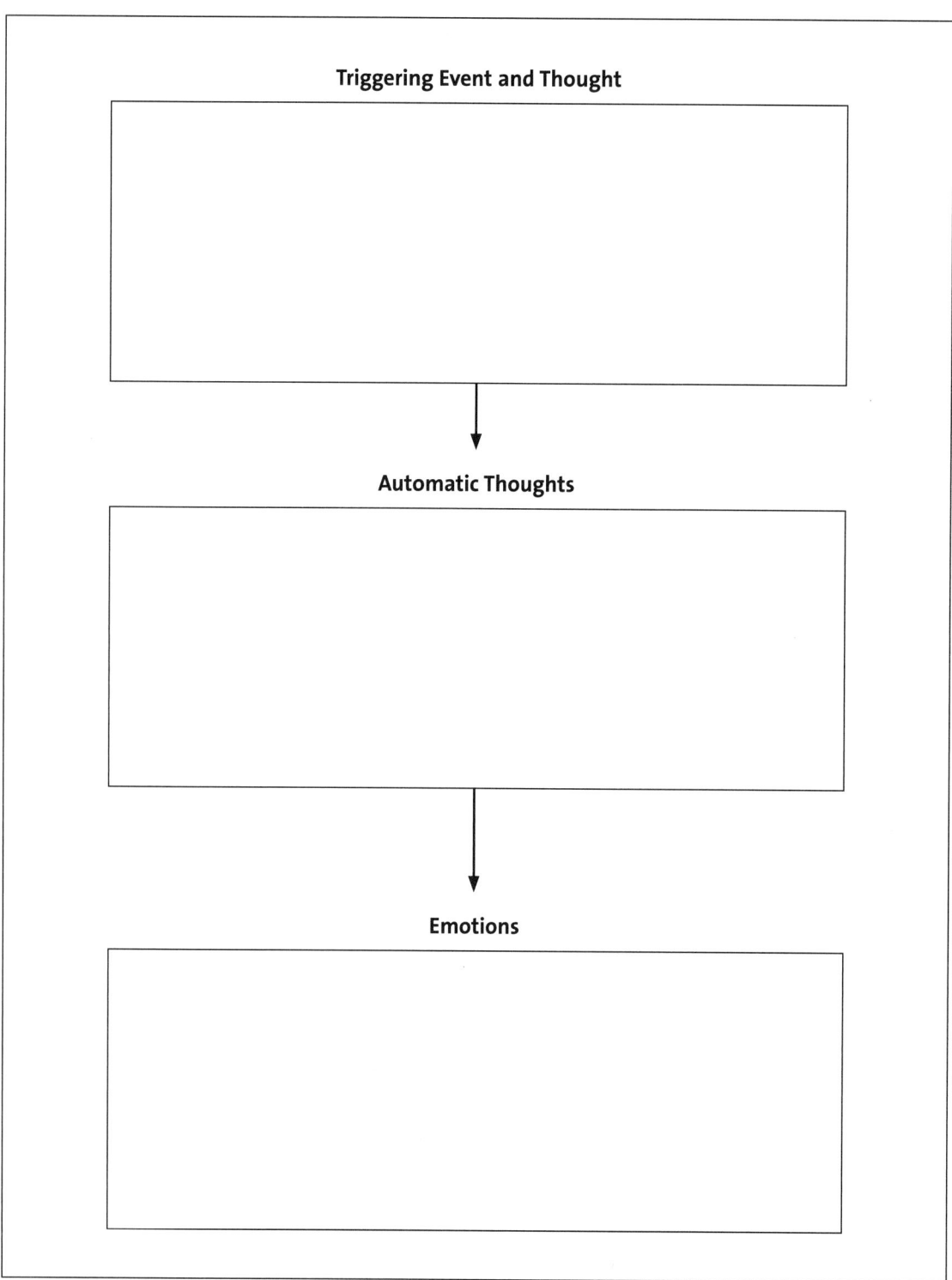

Values

- Achievement
- Adaptability
- Ambition
- Appearance
- Art/Artistic
- Autonomy
- Adventure
- Advocacy
- Courage
- Dependability
- Education
- Entertainment
- Empathy
- Family
- Financial success
- Friendship
- Frugality
- Generosity
- Growth
- Happiness
- Health
- Honesty
- Humor
- Imagination
- Independence
- Integrity
- Intimacy
- Intelligence
- Kindness
- Loyalty
- Openness
- Passion
- Productivity
- Professional success
- Romantic relationships
- Raising children
- Social success (e.g., being known, widely accepted)
- Social responsibility (e.g., giving to community, society, helping others)
- Spirituality
- Tolerance
- Wealth
- Wisdom

My Core Values

1. First, make a list of your core values using the list above or feel free to use your own.

Core values	Importance of values	Percentage of time spent

2. Look at your list above and decide the importance of each value by assigning it a percentage out of a 100. The total sum should not be more than 100.
3. Next, diagram the values on a pie chart and label it "Desired Values."
4. Go back to your list of values and identify how much time you actually devote to each during the week by assigning it a percentage out of a 100. The total sum should not be more than 100.
5. Draw a second pie chart diagram and label it "Time Spent on Values"
6. Discuss ways in which you can make the two diagrams match so that you spend more time on your desired values.

Desired Values Versus Time Spent on Values

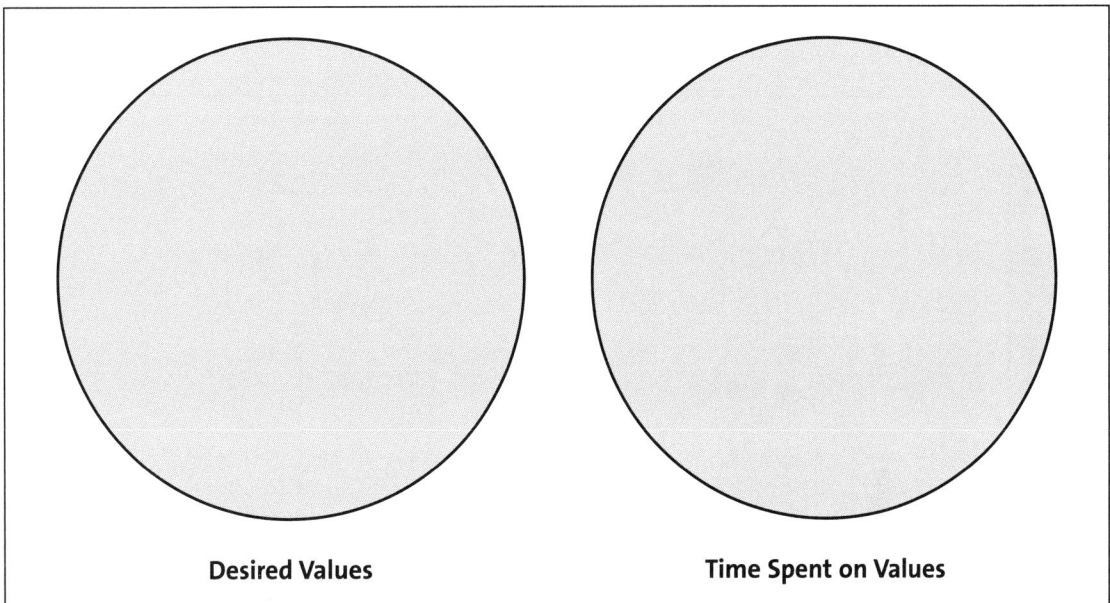

Compulsive, Safety-Seeking, and Avoidance Behaviors

Compulsive Behaviors (e.g., mirror checking, exercising, comparing to others, seeking reassurance, makeup or grooming routine, changing outfits, shaving, skin picking, researching surgery or other appearance-improving methods, skin picking)

Behavior	How often? (Be specific in hours a day, times a day or week)

Safety-Seeking Behaviors (camouflaging with hats, DIY surgery, specific clothing, scarves, sunglasses, altering posture, covering or hiding with your hand, teeth whitening)

Behavior	Degree of use (Always, half the time, or sometimes)

Activities and Situations Avoided (parties, stores, work, leisure, school)

Situation	Degree of avoidance (Always, half the time, or sometimes)

Exposure Hierarchy

Feared or Avoided Situation   **Level of Distress**

_____   _____

_____   _____

_____   _____

_____   _____

_____   _____

_____   _____

_____   _____

_____   _____

_____   _____

_____   _____

_____   _____

_____   _____

_____   _____

_____   _____

_____   _____

_____   _____

_____   _____

_____   _____

_____   _____

_____   _____

Holistic Perceptual Retraining

Training Exercise 1

The goal of this exercise is to demonstrate how detail focus alters one's perceptual experience of visual stimuli.

1. Choose detailed photographs or images unfamiliar to the patient, such as a full bookcase, a painting, a landscape photograph, or an image of an object similar in detail.
2. Ask the patient to list all of the things they notice in the image. Encourage them to list objects, size, shape, and colors present in the image.
3. Ask the patient to rate the image on a scale of 1 to 10, with 1 being unpleasant or unattractive, 5 being neutral, and 10 being very pleasant.
4. Instruct the patient to focus on one particular aspect of the image – for example, a particular book, a branch of a tree, or a small detail in the painting such as the hand of a person in a portrait.
5. Ask the patient to stare at that one small area for a full minute.
6. Take the image away for a period and do not discuss it further. Perhaps review therapy homework during that time in-session.
7. Reintroduce the same image 15 minutes later. What do they notice now? What aspect of the image first drew their visual attention? Was it the area they had been instructed to stare at before? How did their experience of the image change after focusing on the detail? In other words, did they experience the image as pleasant, neutral, or unpleasant? Use the scale of 1–10 as you did initially.
8. Repeat with multiple images over a couple of sessions.
9. Tie in this exercise to their perception in the mirror (how does repeated examination and focus on details alter their overall opinion and experience of an image?).
10. Reinforce psychoeducation of visual processing in BDD

Training Exercise 2

Exercise 1 can be repeated in a somewhat different form by choosing a couple of images with actual slight imperfections, such as a crooked book, imperfect brush stroke, or dead leaf on a tree.

1. Ask the patient to first look at the full image and rate their opinion of it on a scale of 1 to 10, with 1 being an unpleasant image, 5 being neutral, and 10 being a very pleasant image.
2. Now draw their attention to the slight imperfection and ask them to stare at it for a minute.
3. Take the image away and move on to other agenda items in-session. Do not discuss the image.
4. Reintroduce the same image 15 minutes later. What do they notice now? What aspect of the image first drew their visual attention? Was it the area they had been instructed to stare at before? How did their experience of the image change after focusing on the detail?
5. Repeat with multiple images over a couple of sessions.
6. Reflect on how focusing on certain areas of a visual image alters one's overall opinion of it.

Maintenance and Relapse Prevention Plan

The most important reasons I want to maintain my gains

_____

_____

The rational coping statements that help me the most

_____

_____

Treatment techniques and coping strategies that help me the most

_____

_____

My support system: Whom can I turn to for support and how can others help me?

_____

_____

What are my triggers? (what makes my BDD worse – e.g., staying home, not getting enough sleep)

_____

_____

What are some warning signs that my BDD is worsening? (e.g., I start to isolate, I mirror check in the evening)

_____

_____

Self-guided exposure exercises to continue practicing (what is my specific plan on how often, when, and where I will practice)

_____

_____

Short- and Long-Term Life Goals

Three-month goals and some actions I can take

_____

_____

_____

_____

Six-month goals and some actions I can take

_____

_____

_____

_____

One-year goals and some actions I can take

_____

_____

_____

_____

Longer-term goals and some actions I can take

_____

_____

_____

_____

Positive CBT: focusing on building what's right, not on reducing what is wrong

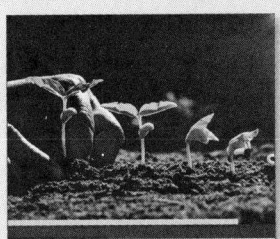

Fredrike Bannink / Nicole Geschwind
Positive CBT
Individual and Group Treatment Protocols for Positive Cognitive Behavioral Therapy

2021, viii + 144 pp., incl. online materials for download
US $49.80 / € 43.95
ISBN 978-0-88937-578-9
Also available as eBook

Positive CBT integrates positive psychology and solution-focused brief therapy within a cognitive-behavioral framework. It focuses on building what is right, rather than on reducing what is wrong. This fourth wave of CBT, developed by Fredrike Bannink, is now being applied worldwide for various psychological disorders. After an introductory chapter exploring the three approaches incorporated in positive CBT, the research into the individual treatment protocol for use with clients with depression by Nicole Geschwind and her colleagues at Maastricht University is presented.

The two 8-session treatment protocols provide practitioners with a step-by-step guide on how to apply positive CBT with individual clients and groups. This approach goes beyond simply symptom reduction and instead focuses on the client's desired future, on finding exceptions to problems and identifying competencies. Topics such as self-compassion, optimism, gratitude, and behavior maintenance are explored.

In addition to the protocols, two workbooks for clients are available online for download by practitioners. The materials for this book can be downloaded from the Hogrefe website after registration.

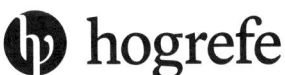

www.hogrefe.com

Advances in Psychotherapy
Evidence-Based Practice

Developed and edited with the support of the Society of Clinical Psychology (APA Division 12)

- Authoritative
- Evidence-Based
- Practice-Oriented
- Easy-to-Read
- Compact
- Inexpensive

Editor-in-chief
Danny Wedding, PhD, MPH

Associate editors
Jonathan S. Comer, PhD
Linda Carter Sobell, PhD, ABPP
Kenneth E. Freedland, PhD
J. Kim Penberthy, PhD, ABPP

Latest releases

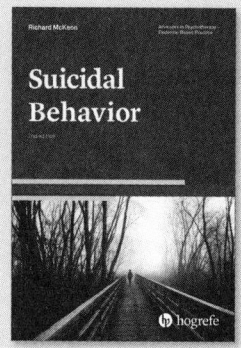
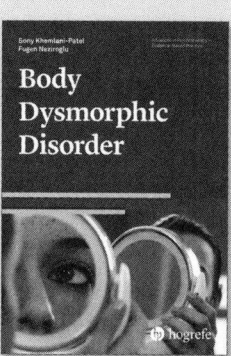
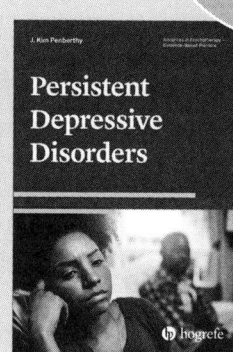
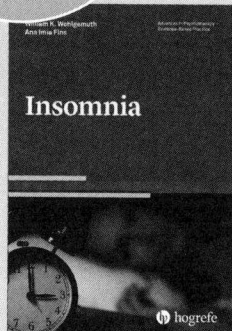

Volume 14, 2nd ed.
ISBN 978-0-88937-506-2

Volume 44
ISBN 978-0-88937-500-0

Volume 43
ISBN 978-0-88937-505-5

Volume 42
ISBN 978-0-88937-415-7

www.hogrefe.com

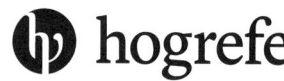

Advances in Psychotherapy
Evidence-Based Practice

All volumes of the series at a glance

Alcohol Use Disorders (Vol. 10)
Alzheimer's Disease and Dementia (Vol. 38)
ADHD in Adults (Vol. 35)
ADHD in Children and Adolescents (Vol. 33)
Autism Spectrum Disorder (Vol. 29)
Binge Drinking and Alcohol Misuse Among College Students and Young Adults (Vol. 32)
Bipolar Disorder (Vol. 1, 2nd ed.)
Body Dysmorphic Disorder (Vol. 44)
Childhood Maltreatment (Vol. 4, 2nd ed.)
Childhood Obesity (Vol. 39)
Chronic Illness in Children and Adolescents (Vol. 9)
Chronic Pain (Vol. 11)
Depression (Vol. 18)
Eating Disorders (Vol. 13)
Elimination Disorders in Children and Adolescents (Vol. 16)
Generalized Anxiety Disorder (Vol. 24)
Growing Up with Domestic Violence (Vol. 23)
Headache (Vol. 30)
Heart Disease (Vol. 2)
Hoarding Disorder (Vol. 40)
Hypochondriasis and Health Anxiety (Vol. 19)
Insomnia (Vol. 42)

Internet Addiction (Vol. 41)
Language Disorders in Children and Adolescents (Vol. 28)
Mindfulness (Vol. 37)
Multiple Sclerosis (Vol. 36)
Nicotine and Tobacco Dependence (Vol. 21)
Nonsuicidal Self-Injury (Vol. 22)
Obsessive-Compulsive Disorder in Adults (Vol. 31)
Persistent Depressive Disorders (Vol. 43)
Phobic and Anxiety Disorders in Children and Adolescents (Vol. 27)
Problem and Pathological Gambling (Vol. 8)
Public Health Tools for Practicing Psychologists (Vol. 20)
Sexual Dysfunction in Women (Vol. 25)
Sexual Dysfunction in Men (Vol. 26)
Sexual Violence (Vol. 17)
Social Anxiety Disorder (Vol. 12)
Substance Use Problems (Vol. 15, 2nd ed.)
Suicidal Behavior (Vol. 14, 2nd ed.)
The Schizophrenia Spectrum (Vol. 5, 2nd ed.)
Treating Victims of Mass Disaster and Terrorism (Vol. 6)
Women and Drinking: Preventing Alcohol-Exposed Pregnancies (Vol. 34)

Coming soon

Affirmative Counseling for Transgender and Gender Diverse Clients
Borderline Personality Disorders

Bullying and Peer Victimization
Psychological Approaches to Cancer Care

Visit **hogrefe.com/us/apt** to get more information about the series!
Prices: US $29.80 / € 24.95 per volume. Standing order price US $24.80 / € 19.95 per volume (minimum 4 successive volumes) + postage & handling. Special rates for APA Division 12 and Division 42 members

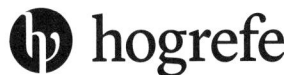

www.hogrefe.com